The Eight-Step Approach to Student Clinical Success

Second Edition

NEW TOOLS FOR PRIORITIZATION!

Lydia R. Zager, MSN, RN, NEA-BC
Co-Executive Director
Leading Learning, LLC
Educational Consultant
Clinical Professor Emerita
College of Nursing
University of South Carolina
Columbia, South Carolina

Loretta Manning, MSN, RN, GNP
President
I CAN Publishing®, Inc.
Co-Executive Director
Leading Learning, LLC
Educational Consultant
Duluth, Georgia

JoAnne Herman, PhD, RN
Professor Emerita
College of Nursing
University of South Carolina
Columbia, South Carolina

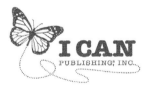

I CAN Publishing®, Inc. ◆ Duluth, GA
www.icanpublishing.com

ISBN: 978-0-9903542-6-0
Library of Congress Control Number: 2018935482
Printed in the United States of America
Second Edition

Copies of this book may be obtained from:

I CAN Publishing®, Inc.
2650 Main Street NW, Suite 100
Duluth, GA 30097
770-495-2488
www.icanpublishing.com

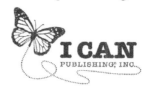

Cover Design: Teresa R. Davidson, Greensboro, NC
Interior Design: Mary Jo Zazueta, Grand Rapids, MI
Publishing Service Manager: Jennifer Robinson, Duluth, GA

Contents

Contributors		*vii*
Preface		*ix*
Acknowledgments		*xi*

CHAPTER 1 **CLINICAL LEARNING: HOW DO I START?** 1

Assess Your Readiness to Be a Clinical Nursing Student 1

Discover How You, as a Novice Student, Think and Learn 1

How Generational Characteristics Can Affect my Learning 3

Appendix A *Clinical Self-Assessment Questionnaire* 5

Appendix B *Interactive Clinical Learning Strategies* 7

Engaging the Learner Activities 9

CHAPTER 2 **LEARN HOW TO STRUCTURE THE CLINICAL DAY** 11

Structure the Clinical Day 11

Structure and Organize Clinical Findings 12

Structure Medication Administration 12

Structure SBAR for Different Scenarios 13

Appendix A *How to Structure a Typical Clinical Day* 14

Appendix B *Typical Day Schedule: A Student guide* 18

Appendix C *Template of Typical Day Schedule: A Student Guide* 19

Appendix D *Shift Report Using SBAR Format* 20

Appendix E *Medication Administration Protocol: A Safe Approach* 21

Appendix F *Example of SBAR Report for Patient Handoff at Change of Shift* 22

Appendix G   *Preparing an SBAR for Call to Healthcare Provider Exercise*   *23*

Appendix H   *Example of SBAR Format to Make a Call to the Healthcare Provider*   *24*

Engaging the Learner Activities   *25*

CHAPTER 3   **IMPROVING CLINICAL DECISION MAKING**   **27**

Develop Prioritization Strategies   27

Comparison of Basic Clinical Assessments with Trending for Potential Complications   28

Apply Inquiry Questions   30

Types of Inquiry Questions   31

Apply Reflection Questions   31

Use Thinking Strategies for Clinical Decision Making   31

Appendix A   *"SAFETY" Model*   *32*

Appendix B   *SAFETY: A New Systematic Approach to Prioritize Nursing Care Based on Standards*   *33*

Appendix C   *The Quick Approach: Inquiry Questions for Classroom and Clinical Knowledge Organized Around the "SAFETY" model*   *34*

Appendix D   *Example of Reflection Questions*   *41*

Appendix E   *Urinary Catheterization Algorithm*   *42*

Appendix F   *Procedure Algorithm Template*   *43*

Appendix G   *Thinking Strategies to Improve Students' Clinical Decision Making*   *44*

Engaging the Learner Activities   *46*

CHAPTER 4   **THE CONCEPT MAP**   **47**

How to Construct and Use a Concept Map   48

Determine Outcomes and Outcome/Evaluation Criteria Table   54

Developing Outcomes and Evaluation Criteria With Interventions   56

Outcome Not Met   57

Outcome Partially Achieved   58

Outcome Achieved   58

Put the Concept Map into Clinical Practice   59

Appendix A   *Example of Adult Health Concept Map*   *61*

Appendix B   *Rubric Grading Tool for Adult Health Concept Map Example*   *63*

Appendix C   *Adult Health Concept Map Tool*   *64*

Appendix D   *AIDES Medication Information Tool*   *66*

Appendix E   *Example of Reflection Questions*   *67*

Appendix F   *History and Pathophysiology Information Tool*   *68*

Appendix G   *Health History and System-Specific Assessment Tool*   *69*

Appendix H   *Lab and Diagnostic Tests and Procedures Tool*   *71*

                 Engaging the Learner Activities   *74*

CHAPTER 5   MASTERING CLINICAL CONCEPTS   75

         Analyze Priority Concepts   75

         Determine Priority Interventions   76

         Evaluate Expected Outcomes   77

         Identify Related Priority Concepts   77

Appendix A   *The Pathophysiology Behind a Decrease in Cardiac/Peripheral Perfusion*   *79*

Appendix B   *Linking Pathophysiology to System-Specific Assessments for Cardiac/Peripheral Perfusion*   *80*

Appendix C   *Linking Pathophysiology to Interventions for Cardiac/ Peripheral Perfusion "PERFUSE"*   *81*

Appendix D   *SAFETY Summary: Concept Cardiac/Peripheral Perfusion*   *82*

Appendix E   *The Pathophysiology Behind Alterations in Oxygenation*   *83*

Appendix F   *Linking Pathophysiology to System-Specific Assessments for Altered Oxygenation*   *84*

Appendix G   *Linking Pathophysiology to First-Do Priority Interventions for Altered Oxygenation*   *85*

Appendix H   *SAFETY Summary: Concept Oxygenation*   *86*

                 Engaging the Learner Activities   *87*

CHAPTER 6   PREPARING FOR SUCCESSFUL SIMULATION   89

         Introduction   89

         Prepare for Simulation   90

Participate in the Simulation   93

Receive and Participate in Debriefing   94

Appendix A   Helpful Tips When Doing Simulation   95

Appendix B   Simulation Preparation Tool ("SAFETY" Tool Adapted
              for Simulation)   96

Appendix C   Example of How to Use the Simulation Preparation Tool   97

              Engaging the Learner Activities   99

CHAPTER 7   EVALUATING CLINICAL PERFORMANCE   101

             Criteria for Clinical Evaluation   101

             Using Feedback Effectively   102

             Participating in the Evaluation Process   104

             STAR Format for Counseling   105

Appendix A   Studying with the "SAFETY" Model   107

Appendix B   Clinical Evaluation Tool   108

Appendix C   Star Counseling Form   112

Appendix D   Example Star Counseling Form   113

             Engaging the Learner Activities   114

CHAPTER 8   LINKING CLINICAL EXPERIENCE TO NCLEX® SUCCESS   115

             Apply NCLEX® Standards Throughout the Clinical Experience   115

             Link the "SAFETY" Model to Clinical Decision Making   116

Appendix A   SAFETY   120

Appendix B   RISK   121

Appendix C   AIDES   122

             Engaging the Learner Activities   123

             REFERENCES   125

             INDEX   129

Contributors

Thank you to our guest author:

Kate K. Chappell, MSN, APRN, CPNP-PC
Clinical Associate Professor
College of Nursing
University of South Carolina
Columbia, South Carolina

Thank you to the following nursing professionals who contributed to this book:

Erin McKinney, MN, RN, RNC-OB
Clinical Professor Emerita
College of Nursing
University of South Carolina
Columbia, South Carolina

Ellen Synovec, MN, RN, NEA-BC
Clinical Professor Emerita
College of Nursing
University of South Carolina
Columbia, South Carolina

Preface

"We often think of nursing as giving meds on time, checking an X-ray to see if the doctor needs to be called or taking an admission at 2:00 a.m. with a smile on our faces. Too often, we forget all the other things that make our job what it truly is: caring and having a desire to make a difference."

~ Erin Pettengill, Missionary Nurse through Mission to the World (MTW)

The time you spend in clinical and simulation is the glue that connects together all that you learn in nursing school. Clinical experiences help integrate what you know while developing competent clinical skills for providing safe and effective care. The expectation for you as new graduate nurses after passing the NCLEX® is to practice as if you have been working for a year!

Prioritization! Decision Making! Clinical Judgment! That is the key for all you do in nursing. You have experienced it with questions on nursing exams, it definitely is on NCLEX®, and it is what clinical is all about, now and when you graduate. We are pleased to include in this second edition of *The Eight-Step Approach to Student Clinical Success*, new prioritization, clinical decision making, and judgment tools to use now and as you transition to a graduate nurse.

Prioritization, decision making, and clinical judgment are also integral parts of simulation. Simulation gives you the opportunity to practice your skills and test your ability to prioritize and make clinical decisions safely. During our consultations and student workshops across the country, there has been an identified need to provide information to guide you as you prepare and participate in simulation. We have a guest author for the chapter, Kate K. Chappell, Clinical Associate Professor, who was a part of the National Council of State Boards of Nursing Simulation Study at the College of Nursing at the University of South Carolina, which was a designated study site. She is an expert in designing and running scenarios and knows how and what you need to prepare for success in simulation.

Engaging the Learner Activities for students is another new feature of this second edition. The activities are included at the end of each chapter. The student-centered learning activities will assist you to engage in your own learning, help you connect classroom to clinical, and link

NCLEX® standards to practice. The activities refer you to the books *Concepts Made Insanely Easy for Clinical Nursing! A New Approach to Prioritizing Clinical Nursing* (Manning & Zager, 2014), and *Medical Surgical Nursing Concepts Made Insanely Easy!* (Manning & Zager, 2014).

The Eight-Step Approach to Student Clinical Success is the answer to the NCSBN's new initiative to expand and optimize the measurement of clinical judgment on the NCLEX-RN® examination. Research from the NCSBN concluded that 50 percent of nurses were involved in errors of nursing in some way, and 65 percent of those errors were a result of poor clinical decision making skills (https://www.ncsbn.org/11436.htm). This book will guide you how to learn to *"Think Like a Nurse"* from your first day as a student nurse throughout your clinical nursing education.

The second edition of *The Eight-Step Approach to Student Clinical Success* continues to honor your requests for a practical, how-to approach for clinical. We dedicate this work to the many student nurses who are constantly striving for an increased level of mastery as a nurse! We wish you much success on your journey!

Acknowledgments

We want to acknowledge and express our appreciation to the clinical faculty at the University of South Carolina in Columbia, South Carolina. We appreciate your contributions, your helpful suggestions, the adaptation and use of many of the forms in this book throughout the clinical courses.

We also want to thank the nursing students across the country for all of the useful feedback that has assisted us throughout the development of the tools and book.

+ We want to thank all of our families for their never-ending support of this project. Their insight, humor, and patience help more than they know, thank you!

+ We want to thank Jennifer Robinson, our Administrative Director, who supports us with all aspects of writing, publishing, and distributing our books and keeps us organized!

+ We want to thank Teresa Davidson, our friend and artist, who takes our ideas and brings them alive in the book covers. Thank you for hanging in with us as we do multiple revisions of the cover up until time to go to print!

+ We want to thank Mary Jo Zazueta, our friend and book designer who always makes our work look good!

+ We want to thank to all of our contributors who add to the quality and usefulness of our book.

+ A special thanks to our guest author, Kate Chappell for her excellent and timely chapter on simulation...well done!

Clinical Learning: How Do I Start?

IN THIS CHAPTER YOU WILL:

→ Assess your readiness to be a successful student

→ Discover how you, as a novice student, think and learn

→ Explore how generational characteristics can affect your learning

---

ASSESS YOUR READINESS TO BE A CLINICAL NURSING STUDENT

As a clinical nursing student, you are preparing for your important new role as a registered nurse. Through a collaborative partnership with your clinical instructor, you can make learning a positive experience that will set the tone for how you approach client care.

Clinical can be a scary process, but not when you are adequately prepared. Through adequate preparation, clinical is extremely rewarding. This chapter will help you assess your readiness for your clinical experience. The **Clinical Self-Assessment Questionnaire** (Appendix A) will help you with this process as you begin your role. If the answer to any of the questions in the questionnaire is "No," the resource column will help you find the information you need.

DISCOVER HOW YOU, AS A NOVICE STUDENT, THINK AND LEARN

The brain is structured in neural networks. Learning is the process of developing new and more complex neural networks. Your learning is enhanced when you are actively engaged in the content through repetition and participate in the experience (Kaufer, 2016). New learning is stored in the brain with very few interconnections to other things you have previously learned. Interconnections are formed through repetition thus connecting the new knowledge to existing knowledge. This is why you may not recall content you have previously learned.

Initial learning is temporary. Repetition is critical for you to learn. Clinical experiences give you the opportunity to practice, practice, practice. The neural networks become better connected through increased repetition. For example, every time you insert a Foley catheter, the relationship among the steps of the procedure, sterile technique, rationale for the Foley, potential complications and priority client teaching increases the strength of the connection of these parts to each other. The more interconnections that are established, the more expertise you develop.

Do you recognize any of these characteristics in yourself?

+ I make decisions quickly before thinking about all the options that are possible. In other words, I will jump to conclusions.

+ I have difficulty applying classroom content to clinical situations.

+ I am easily overwhelmed by data, (i.e., information in the medical record, labs, etc.).

+ I have difficulty distinguishing relevant from irrelevant information.

+ I am sometimes afraid of engaging in a clinical experience that seems challenging.

+ I am often unorganized in my approach to clinical problems.

As novice student learners, you might be apprehensive about clinical experiences. You may see clinical as a set of tasks that must be accomplished. You also may feel that clinical is a test of your personal capabilities. No wonder you feel stressed! The following chapters provide strategies designed to help you progress and provide the tools necessary to be a superior clinical student.

HOW GENERATIONAL CHARACTERISTICS CAN AFFECT MY LEARNING

When you combine the characteristics you have as a novice learner with the characteristics of either Generations X, Y(millennial) or Z, it can make a difference in how you study and learn. Look at the following table. Which generation do you belong to? Do the learning needs describe you?

Learning Needs	Generation X (born after 1965)	Generation Y–Millennials (born after 1980)	Generation Z (born after 1995)
Structure In The Learning Process	• Yes, but like to be creative.	• Yes, very structured.	• Yes, very structured.
Supportive Interactive Relationships	• Yes, but may be skeptical of the instructor. • I am self-reliant and independent.	• Yes, prefer engagement with instructor.	• Yes, prefer engagement with instructor.
How You Want Information	• Tell me only what I need to know. • How the information relates to the real world. • Don't like "touchy feely" activities.	• Hands on/interactive experience. • Like to be creative, use trial and error. • Like visual aids. • Have a short attention span.	• Communicate with images, 5 words or less. • Want information instantaneously and I lose interest quickly. • Want faculty to be prepared.
Group Work	• Yes.	• Yes.	• Yes.
Feedback	• Straight forward, immediate feedback.	• Daily, but do not like negative feedback.	• Constant and immediate.
Comfortable With Technology	• I'm technologically, savvy.	• Yes, expect technology to be a part of the learning experience.	• Like technology, but also want an instructor who keeps me engaged.

You are most likely technologically savvy and are used to multi-tasking—talking on the cell phone while working on the computer, and doing your homework. However, it is impossible to think about more than one thing at a time. In fact, what you do is toggle back and forth between the subjects. The danger is that it can be very difficult to learn anything in depth, which is essential when you are learning to critically think in order to make appropriate clinical decisions.

There are some strategies that can help you be successful as a novice multi-generational learner. The word **COACH** can help you remember how to be successful!

C – Collaborate and Create Partnerships
With your clinical instructor and peers

O – Off with the Toggle Switch
Don't multi-task when you are trying to learn

A – Acquire Basic Knowledge
Only you can learn the required information

C – Communicate
With your instructor, peers, and clients

H – Have to be Receptive to Feedback
Be willing to make changes

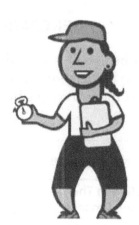

The **Interactive Clinical Learning Strategies** (Appendix B) may be used by your instructor during clinical, clinical lab, or during simulation. You can also use them while you are studying with your fellow students to reinforce your learning and preparedness for clinical.

Now you are ready to complete the **Clinical Self-Assessment Questionnaire** (Appendix A) and get started! The following chapters in this book will give you the guidance and information you need to be a successful student in clinical, the learning lab, and during simulation!

CLINICAL SELF-ASSESSMENT QUESTIONNAIRE

Self-Assessment Questions	Yes, I Know	No, I Need Help	Resources: Where to Find Help
1. Do I understand the expected outcomes of this clinical?			Refer to your course syllabus and clinical instructor.
2. Do I have the knowledge, skills, and abilities to provide safe and effective care?			1. Refer to course textbooks. 2. Reflect on prior clinical experiences with similar types of clients. 3. Work with other students in your clinical group.
3. Do I know the policies and procedures, medication system/protocols, documentation process, supply systems, and safety or quality assurance concerns?			1. Review unit and clinical facilitiy's policies and procedures. 2. Learn the medication system/protocols for the unit, the documentation process, and supply systems.
4. Do I know how to prepare for my clinical experience?			Refer to Chapter 2

5. Do I know how to structure my clinical day? This includes:
  a. Orientation to the unit
  b. Clinical day routine
  c. Documentation
  d. Medication administration
  e. Written plans for care (i.e., your concept map)
  f. Prepare and give SBAR reports
  g. Pre – post conferences
			Refer to Chapter 2, 3

6. Do I know what thinking strategies I can use to improve my clinical reasoning?			Refer to Chapter 1, 2, 3, 5
7. Do I know how to use NCLEX® activities to organize my learning?			Refer to Chapter 8

cont'd on next page

APPENDIX A

CLINICAL SELF-ASSESSMENT QUESTIONNAIRE *(cont'd)*

Self-Assessment Questions	Yes, I Know	No, I Need Help	Resources: Where to Find Help
8. Do I know how to answer inquiry and reflection questions?			Refer to Chapter 3, 5
9. Do I know how to use a concept map in clinical?			Refer to Chapter 4
10. Do I know how to make clinical judgments through the use of thinking strategies?			Refer to Chapter 3, 5
11. Do I know how to prepare, perform, and how I will be evaluated when I am in simulation for my clinical experience?			Refer to Chapter 6
12. Do I know how to receive formal and informal feedback?			Refer to Chapter 7
13. Do I know how performance counseling will be used to help me improve my clinical practice and to notify me if I am not meeting clinical requirements?			Refer to Chapter 7
14. Do I know what the evaluation criteria are that I must meet to be successful?			Refer to Chapter 7

INTERACTIVE CLINICAL LEARNING STRATEGIES

Game	Description	Use
Scavenger Hunt	• Work in groups of 2 or 3. • Locate items on the unit and describe their exact location. • Each group will take the others to the location.	• Helpful during clinical and simulation orientation to identify location of essential equipment, supplies.
Skill Day	• A planned clinical day for clinical skill reinforcement (Refer to Chapter 6).	• Can use early each semester to review new, previously learned and/or practice clinical skills.
Infection Control Day	• A planned day in the lab for you to identify for each client, the appropriate personal protective equipment (PPE) that would need to be used in the care of the client (i.e., you will be given a card to give an IM injection and must select the correct PPE, etc.).	• Assists in reinforcing infection control application that is very difficult for students to master. • These are important safety and NCLEX® Standards.
Clinical Scene Investigation— CSI	• Identify a mystery, unknown clinical fact, and/or dilemma such as "why is the client suddenly itching?" • Generate a list of possible explanations, such as drug-drug interactions, allergy, contact dermatitis, etc. • Next investigate the different explanations with your fellow students until you arrive at a conclusion, or realize you do not have enough data to solve the mystery.	• Helps you seek out needed information. • Helpful tool for group learning. • (Hint: This is a great strategy when you do not know the answer!)
Deck of Doom	• Card game that reviews a clinical situation on a card. • Your instructor or a fellow student will give you a card. • Answer questions and report back to the group at post-conference. • An example may include the following: The client's blood sugar at 1 PM is 47 mg/dL; what are the priority nursing interventions for this client?	• Post-conference game, or to be used for fun during the clinical day. • Used to reinforce learning, such as hard-to-remember concepts, like the onset, peak times of different insulins. • Use in the classroom for new information or test review.

cont'd on next page

INTERACTIVE CLINICAL LEARNING STRATEGIES *(cont'd)*

Game	Description	Use
Leading Learning for the Day	• Work together in pairs or with a group based on your instructor's instructions.	• Helps you build confidence. • Helps you develop leadership, team building and collaboration skills.
War Stories	• Clinical instructors or students share clinical experiences that can be positive or negative or even funny. • Who can tell the best story?	• Helps you make connections between reality-based practice with theoretical learning. • Stories are a vivid personal teaching method that help you connect to clinical. • Stories may involve both positive and negative clinical experiences.
Who Wants to be a Super Nurse?	• The clinical instructor may ask questions in your group about information you are expected to know. You will have a choice of life lines to answer the question. • You can answer the question yourself. • You can ask another student, (call a friend). • You can ask the group, (poll the audience) and choose to agree or disagree with the answer.	• This helps you to reinforce learning.

ENGAGING THE LEARNER ACTIVITIES

STUDENT-CENTERED LEARNING ACTIVITIES
LINKED TO PROFESSIONAL AND NCLEX® STANDARDS

Resources Needed for Activity	*The Eight-Step Approach for Student Clinical Success* (Zager, Manning & Herman, 2018)
Standards	**Student Instructions**

Management of Care
 	
Recognize limitations of self and others and seek assistance.
	Self-Assessment Questionnaire
	(Refer to Appendix A)
	
	1. Complete the Self-Assessment questionnaire.
	  a. Identify your greatest challenges.
	  b. Identify your strengths.
	  c. Share ideas about what you can do to prepare for clinical (i.e., resources, references, etc.).
	  d. Identify specific learning goals for yourself.

Management of Care Organize workload to manage time effectively.	**Scavenger Hunt** (Refer to the Scavenger Hunt in Appendix B) 2. Look for the items given to you by your instructor for the Scavenger Hunt and document where they are located on your assigned unit.

Assessing Your Learning Style	**Characteristics of Novice and Multi-Generational Learner**
	(Refer to Chapter 1)
	
	3. Review in Chapter 1 the characteristics of a novice and multi-generational learner.
	  a. Identify characteristics of a novice learner that apply to you.
	  b. Identify which generational characteristics apply to you.
	  c. Identify strategies that can help you be successful in your learning.

NOTES

Learn How to Structure the Clinical Day

IN THIS CHAPTER YOU WILL LEARN HOW TO:

- ➤ Structure the clinical day
- ➤ Structure and organize clinical findings
- ➤ Structure medication administration
- ➤ Structure SBAR for different scenarios

STRUCTURE THE CLINICAL DAY

Do you ever feel overwhelmed with how to organize a clinical day? Do you ever experience a sleepless night before clinical worrying about administering multiple medications? Our goal is to provide you with tools and a structure to assist in planning and organizing the clinical day.

Effective communication with the nursing staff can make all the difference in the quality of your clinical experience. Discuss with your clinical instructor the skills and procedures that can be done alone, with the nursing staff, or your instructor. Determine how you will communicate. Coordinate with the staff your clinical assignment and aspects of the care you will be performing.

The next step is to plan your clinical day. **How to Structure a Typical Clinical Day** (Appendix A) provides you an example of how to plan your day. The structure can be adapted to any clinical setting, and it will help decrease your anxiety and optimize your learning experience. It may seem like a lot of work, but the time spent in planning will help ensure your success.

STRUCTURE AND ORGANIZE CLINICAL FINDINGS

You may feel overwhelmed and unsure about how to organize the information you get from report, orders for procedures and medications, and the client's medical record. Without a structured format, it is easy to be disorganized in thinking, delivery of care, and timeliness. This disorganization makes it difficult for you to document accurately. In this chapter, we have included an example of a **Typical Clinical Day Schedule: A Student Guide** (Appendix B) and a blank **Typical Clinical Day Schedule: A Student Guide Template** (Appendix C) for you to use and adapt to organize your clinical day schedule. Also included is an example of a **Shift Report Using SBAR Format** (Appendix D) that is very helpful to organize your clinical information to give an effective and accurate report.

STRUCTURE MEDICATION ADMINISTRATION

The **Medication Administration Protocol: A Safe Approach** (Appendix E) is a way for you to develop a safe medication practice essential to help prevent medication errors. Adverse drug events, harm caused by medication errors, affects approximately 5% of hospitalized clients. It is the most common type of inpatient error (Agency for Healthcare Research and Quality, 2015). Multiple federal agencies such as Agency for Healthcare Research and Quality (AHRQ), Institute for Safe Medication (ISMP), Quality and Safety Education for Nurses (QSEN), etc. have developed guidelines designed to decrease medication errors. These guidelines include recommendations such as establishing a no-interruption zone and using a structured checklist for medication administration that includes supplies and clinical information you need prior to giving medications (Beyea, 2014).

The **Medication Administration Protocol: A Safe Approach** (Appendix E) incorporates the recommended national guidelines that will assist you to develop a safe habit for administering medications. This habit will help you feel confident that you are prepared to give your medications. In order for the medication protocol to become a habit, you must use it in all of your clinical courses. This repetition strengthens your habits of safe medication administration.

STRUCTURE SBAR FOR DIFFERENT SCENARIOS

The SBAR structure is a formal method of communicating vital patient information to your peers, the charge nurse, and healthcare providers during change of shift report, phone calls or transfer of clients between units, or other facilities. It was developed to improve patient safety. **SBAR** stands for **Situation-Background-Assessment-Recommendation** (Institute for Healthcare Improvement, 2018).

S – **Situation** includes a clear and concise description of the situation and/or problem, (i.e., the client presented with a new onset of confusion and combativeness).

B – **Background** includes relevant background information that relates to the client's current situation, (i.e., client's current diagnoses, past medical history, healthcare providers and current medications).

A – **Assessment** includes your current system-specific assessment and analysis of results.

R – **Recommendation** includes what do you currently need to clarify, report for follow-up or need from the healthcare provider. (Institute for Healthcare Improvement, 2018).

An **Example of SBAR Report For Patient Handoff At Change Of Shift** (Appendix F) is an example of what should be included. **Preparing a SBAR For Call To Healthcare Provider Exercise** (Appendix G) is an exercise for you to practice how to prepare a SBAR from your change of shift report and in preparation for calling the healthcare provider for change in client status, or need for new orders, etc. **Example of SBAR Format To Make A Call To The Healthcare Provider** (Appendix H) is an example, so you can compare how you did on your SBAR report you completed as compared to the example in Appendix F.

The tools described and included in the appendices will help you organize your clinical day, document with accuracy, administer medications, give an accurate report and ultimately provide safe and effective care for your clients.

APPENDIX A

HOW TO STRUCTURE A TYPICAL CLINICAL DAY
Adapt to fit the schedule for your clinical day.

Time	Student Activity	Information About Your Client
6:45 AM Prior to pre-conference	Get report (SBAR) from your nurse. Check for: • New orders. • New medications. • Time of 1st medication. • Check if NPO for tests, surgery or procedures. If so, will they get any of their medications (i.e., insulin, antihypertensives, etc.)?	
Pre-conference	Review your clinical concept maps and plans for the day with your instructor.	
7:00 – 7:20 AM	See your client for a quick assessment: • Respiratory status, in pain, safety issues, etc. • Check IVs. Make sure they are patent and running at the right rate with the right fluid. • Check for any other lines, tubes, tube patency, and/or drainage. • Take client's BP and pulse. • Check on blood sugars and/or obtain glucometer reading. • Administer insulin or other before meals medications. • Always check to see if the medication has been given, is being held, etc. • Prepare for any scheduled tests.	

HOW TO STRUCTURE A TYPICAL CLINICAL DAY *(cont'd)*
Adapt to fit the schedule for your clinical day.

Time	Student Activity	Information About Your Client
8:00 – 9:30 AM	• Give AM medications. • Perform other client procedures as ordered. • Prepare client for scheduled procedures/ surgery if scheduled. • Complete focused system-specific assessment. • Note any trending of clinical findings that could indicate potential complications. • Document findings, inform instructor and nursing staff of any concerns. • Complete or ensure AM care is done (often a good time to do the assessment).	
9:30 – 10 AM	• First-documentation entered to include assessments and other findings. • Implement and evaluate your priority nursing interventions (i.e., coughing and deep breathing, etc.). • "MOVE Your Client"–Ambulate, get them up in chair or turn (as condition allows); assess client's activity tolerance and document (Manning, L. & Zager, L. 2014, p. 146).	
10:30 AM	• Continue to assess client and document. • Evaluate response to PRN medications. • Complete any treatments or procedures as ordered (this may be earlier in your day, depending on the time of the test). • Complete client teaching and document. • Continue to check for new healthcare provider's orders. • Check for lab result (i.e., PTT and INR if on heparin, etc.).	

cont'd on next page

APPENDIX A

HOW TO STRUCTURE A TYPICAL CLINICAL DAY *(cont'd)*
Adapt to fit the schedule for your clinical day.

Time	Student Activity	Information About Your Client
11:00 – 12:00	• Give medications as ordered. • Assist with meals as needed. • Assess vital signs as ordered. • Continue to assess client and document findings. • Assess and provide care for indwelling lines, peg tubes, etc. • Continue interventions and assess effectiveness.	
Lunch	• Plan your lunch around your client's needs (you will need to cover for your fellow students).	
1:00 – 1:45 PM	• Continue to assess if desired client outcomes are being met and documented. • Are there any trending concerns in the client's assessment findings? If so, report to your instructor and the client's nurse. • Continue client teaching and document. • Complete any scheduled interventions or procedures.	
1:45 – 2:30 PM	• Complete final assessment and document client's progress toward desired outcomes. • Document I & O (i.e., IV or PO intake, NG tube or Foley output, etc.). • Make sure client is safe (i.e. ,bed rails up, bed alarms in place, etc.). • Ensure the client's room is neat. • Check to see if all medications have been given and documented with client responses	

HOW TO STRUCTURE A TYPICAL CLINICAL DAY *(cont'd)*
Adapt to fit the schedule for your clinical day.

Time	Student Activity	Information About Your Client
2:30 PM	Give SBAR to the assigned nurse.	
2:30 – 3:00 PM	Attend post-conference.	
HOME	Go home, kick your feet up and be happy another clinical day is over! Seriously though, take time to reflect on how the day went, what went well, and what you can do to improve your next clinical day.	

APPENDIX B

TYPICAL DAY SCHEDULE: A STUDENT GUIDE
(May vary per clinical and client needs.)

When you arrive, before 6:45 AM

+ Get report from your nurse.

+ Check for new orders, new meds, time of first med, check if NPO for test, which meds are they getting, AM blood sugars.

7:00 – 7:20 AM Pre-conference

+ Assess client's BP and pulse.

+ Give 7:30 medications, insulin (check to see if it has been given).

+ See your client and assess quickly, check IVs, make sure they are patent and running at the right rate with the right fluid, check for any other lines, tubes that they are patent and what is draining.

By 9:30 AM

+ Give medications and complete assessment or vice versa as appropriate.

+ Enter your assessment findings in the documentation system per protocol.

+ Give AM care (a great time to do or complete your client's assessment).

10 AM

+ Document opening nursing note with AM assessment by_____(Time).

10:30 AM

+ Treatments or procedures ordered (this may come earlier if scheduled for tests).

+ Implement client teaching as needed. Continue to check for new orders from healthcare provider.

+ Check for lab results, (i.e., PTT & INR if on heparin, blood sugar if on insulin, etc.). 11:00–12:00 check for noon blood sugar if ordered, eat lunch, feed client if needed.

11 AM

+ Document vital signs, note any trending that could indicate potential complication. Continue to assess client's response and progress toward expected outcomes.

Lunch for 30 min between the hours of 11:00 and 12:00 based on your client's needs. Coordinate with other students.

Give 11 and 12 o'clock meds if ordered, flush Intermittent Access Venous Device per protocol

+ Continue to reinforce client teaching and interventions to help your client achieve the expected outcomes and continuously reassess your client.

1:00 PM

+ Wrap-up, do final assessment, make sure the client is safe, needs are met, and the room is neat and free of clutter.

+ Complete I & O, document per protocol. Check to see that all medications have been given and documented.

1:30 PM

+ Document your final notes: include evaluation of your client's progress or lack of progress toward the expected outcomes.

+ Is your client getting better? Include I & O. Document information as appropriate on IV flow rates, insertion sites, drains, dressings, etc. Document client teaching and evaluation of client's level of understanding.

By 2:00 PM

+ Report off to your nurse and your clinical instructor using SBAR.

2:00 PM Post-conference

TEMPLATE OF TYPICAL DAY SCHEDULE: A STUDENT GUIDE
(May vary per clinical and client needs.)

Time: _____ (When you arrive)

✦ Get report from your nurse.

✦ Check for new orders, new meds, time of first med, check if NPO for test, which meds are they getting, AM blood sugars.

Time: _____ (Pre-conference)

✦ Assess client's BP and pulse.

✦ Give ordered medications, insulin (check to see if it has been given).

✦ See your client and assess quickly, check IVs, make sure they are patent and running at the right rate with the right fluid, check for any other lines, tubes that they are patent and what is draining.

Time: _____ (Within two hours of starting your clinical)

✦ Give medications and complete assessment or vice versa as appropriate.

✦ Enter your assessment findings in the documentation system per protocol.

✦ Give AM/PM care as appropriate (a great time to do or complete your client's assessment).

✦ Document opening nursing note with assessment by _____ (Time).

Time: _____ (Within third hour of your clinical)

✦ Treatments or procedures ordered (this may come earlier if scheduled for tests).

✦ Implement client teaching as needed. Continue to check for new orders from healthcare provider.

✦ Check for lab results, (i.e., PTT & INR if on heparin, blood sugar if on insulin, etc.). Check for blood sugar if ordered, eat, feed client if needed.

✦ Document vital signs, note any trending that could indicate potential complication. Continue to assess client's response and progress toward expected outcomes.

Mealtime for 30 min. (Between the hours of _____ based on your client's needs. Coordinate with other students.)

Time: _____ (Give other meds if ordered, flush Intermittent Access Venous Device per protocol)

✦ Continue to reinforce client teaching and interventions to help your client achieve the expected outcomes and continuously reassess your client.

Time: _____ (At least one hour prior to departure and post-conference)

✦ Wrap-up, do final assessment, make sure the client is safe, needs are met, and the room is neat and free of clutter.

✦ Complete I & O, document per protocol. Check to see that all medications have been given and documented.

Time: _____ (At least ½ hour prior to departure and post-conference)

✦ Document your final notes: include evaluation of your client's progress or lack of progress toward the expected outcomes.

✦ Is your client getting better? Include I & O. Document information as appropriate on IV flow rates, insertion sites, drains, dressings, etc. Document client teaching and evaluation of client's level of understanding.

Time: _____ (Last 15 minutes prior to departure and post-conference)

✦ Report off to your nurse and your clinical instructor using SBAR.

Time: _____ (Post-conference)

APPENDIX D

SHIFT REPORT USING SBAR FORMAT

The Situation and Background will only need to be entered the first time you report on this client.

Situation: Client Name, Age, Sex, Room Number.

Brief concise report of current situation and/or problem.

Names of healthcare providers.

Background: Admission Diagnosis (date of surgery).

Past medical history that is significant (hypertension, heart failure, etc.).

Known allergies.

Current medications.

Assessment: Code Status, any advance directives, DNR orders, Power of Attorney Health Care (POAHC).

Abnormal vital signs or assessment findings.

Procedures done in previous 24 hours including results/outcomes (include client's post-procedure vitals/assessment).

IV fluids/drips/site; when is site to be changed.

Current pain score—what has been done to manage pain.

Safety needs—fall risk, skin risk, etc.

Recommendations: What are the needed changes in the plan of care (diet, activity, medication, consultations)?

What are you concerned about?

Discharge planning concerns or needs?

Pending labs/x-rays, etc.

Calls made to healthcare provider(s).

What does the next shift or unit need to do or be aware of (i.e., labs to be drawn in AM, etc.).

Please remember to "Repeat back or use the Read back technique" to verify the received information (i.e., orders that include DNR, diagnostic tests, medications, and/or essential components of care, etc.).

MEDICATION ADMINISTRATION PROTOCOL: A SAFE APPROACH

Prior to Beginning Medication Administration

1. Prior to beginning medication administration:
  a. Verify orders.
  b. Gather needed client assessments (i.e., BP, pulse, or other required assessment data).
  c. Check needed lab results (i.e., potassium level if client has furosemide ordered, blood sugar or glucometer readings for insulin, drug levels like digoxin).
  d. Check to see if any clients are NPO, or are going for procedures, dialysis, etc.
  e. Check to see if any medications have Black Box Warnings or are high-alert medications.

2. Pull the Medication Record for your client (the MAR). Do only one client at a time.

3. Know the purpose of each medication. Do you have all the information you need prior to giving the medication? If not, obtain and review this information and have it ready.
  a. Action of the drug.
  b. Key adverse reactions.
  c. Nursing implications.
  d. Why the client is getting the medication. Is the drug appropriate for this client?
  e. Food/drug or drug/drug interactions.
  f. Known allergies.
  g. What do you need to teach your client about the medication? (Manning & Rayfield, 2017)

4. Let your instructor know you are ready to check off your medications.
Preparing Medications for Administration
5. Obtain the medications you need. (Your clinical instructor may have to do this for you based on the medication system in your facility, i.e., Bar Code Scanners, Pyxis, etc.).
6. Have MAR visible and check your medications (i.e., vials, IV piggy backs, IV fluids, etc.) beside the ordered drug on the MAR.

7. Check the medications against the MAR in order as they are listed. Leave medications in packaging and do not draw medications from the vials without your instructor.
  a. Do you have the right medication?
  b. Is the medication scheduled for this time?
  c. Is it the right dose?
  d. Is there any information you need to document prior to giving the medication (i.e., BP readings, digoxin levels, etc.) that you do not have?
  e. Is there any medication that needs to be held or any order that needs to be questioned?
  f. Has the medication already been given?
  g. Based on what you know about the medication, does it make sense (rationale) that this client is getting this medication? (Manning & Rayfield, 2017)

8. With your instructor, prepare the correct dosage (i.e., cut the pill, draw up the correct dose from a vial for IV, IM, subcutaneous injections, etc.).
Administering the Medications
9. Once you have completed the check-off with your instructor, take your MAR and the medications still in their packaging (it may be the Bar Code Scanner or beside medication delivery system) to the client's bedside.
10. Perform seven rights for medications and check your medications with the MAR as you give the medication to the client.
11. Sign off the medications on the MAR or documentation system as the client takes them and answer any client or family questions.
12. Return the MAR to the appropriate place and note when your next medications are due. Document as appropriate.
13. Evaluate client's response to medications per protocol. (Manning & Rayfield, 2017)
14. Document client's response and progress toward outcome.

APPENDIX F

EXAMPLE OF SBAR REPORT FOR PATIENT HANDOFF AT CHANGE OF SHIFT

Setting: 1600 Hours (4 PM) in a small emergency department (ED)

Situation:	James Mulhaney 62-year-old male Client of P. Smith, MD Admitted to ED with new onset of erratic behavior at work
Background:	The client arrived by car at 1500 (3:00 pm), brought by his manager from his job as a cashier/bagger at a grocery store. His manager states, "He was acting really strange, like he was drunk or something. He yelled at a customer to 'leave' and 'quit bothering me' when they asked him to use the bags they brought to the store. He swatted in the air like there was something after him. Then he almost fell down, seemed out of it, so I brought him to ED." His manager reports no knowledge of any past issues with acting erratically. None of the client's family members can be reached via phone. The manager brought the client's last employee health fair form (completed 4 months ago) with him.
Past Medical History:	*(Information from employee health fair form completed 4 months ago):* HTN, treated prostate cancer (3 years ago), smoking X 35 yrs. Blood Pressure—152/80. Blood sugar by finger stick—94 mg/dL. Reported medications—Atenolol 25 mg once daily. Oxybutynin chloride 5 mg twice daily. Aspirin 81 mg once daily.
Allergies:	No known drug allergies (NKDA)
Assessment:	Emergency department nursing assessment: Weight—190 lbs. Finger stick blood sugar done at 1630 (4:30pm)—90 mg/dL. Vital signs 1615 hours (4:15 pm)—T 99.6°F, HR 98 BPM, RR 20/min, BP 140/74. Pulse Ox—94% on room air. Pain score 1615 hours (4:15pm)—FLACC (Face, Legs, Activity, Cry, Consolability) 5 out of 10.
Code Status:	Unknown
Recommendations:	Initial orders by the ED healthcare provider: • Vital signs and mental status checks hourly. • Regular supervision and safety checks. • Strict I and O. • Regular diet. • Encourage fluids. • Check finger stick blood sugar now. • Consult for an acute psychiatric evaluation.

Please remember to "Repeat back or use the Read back technique" to verify the received information (i.e., orders that include DNR, diagnostic tests, medications, and/or essential components of care, etc.).

PREPARING AN SBAR FOR CALL TO HEALTHCARE PROVIDER EXERCISE

Instructions:

- ○ Prepare a SBAR report for a call to the healthcare provider.
- ○ Use the findings (below) from the nursing assessment you completed after you received the **Example of SBAR Report For Patient Handoff At Change Of Shift** (Appendix F) from another nurse at the change of shift.

Assessment:

General Assessment: Client is combative with frequent comments of "leave me alone", "why am I in jail?", and brushing away/swatting away motions. Responses to questions are variable in their match to questions.

Neuro: Oriented X 1 (person only).

Cardiovascular: S_1S_2, no murmurs, gallops, or rubs. Brachial pulses 2+; posterior tibialis pulses 3+. Capillary refill 2 seconds to upper extremities, 3 seconds to lower extremities.

Respiratory: Clear, equal breath sounds bilaterally without apparent distress.

Gastrointestinal (GI): Active bowel sounds, soft rounded abdomen. No tenderness to light palpation.

Genitourinary (GU): No discharge noted. Reports no difficulty with urination. Client voided using urinal, urine pink-tinged with strong odor.

Integumentary: Color pale, skin sweaty.

The on-call psychiatrist reports it will be 2 hours before they can see the client to do their evaluation.

Your clinical judgment based on your assessment findings: You suspect one potential cause of this client's mental status might be a urinary tract infection and you need to inform the healthcare provider and discuss the plan.

Prepare your SBAR report.
Refer to the **Engaging the Learner Activity** at the end of this chapter and
Shift Report Using SBAR Format (Appendix D) as a guide.

When you are done, check how you SBAR report compared to the **Example of a SBAR Format to Make a Call to the Healthcare Provider** (Appendix H)! How did you do? Did you include all of the pertinent information? Did you make recommendations so that you would receive the orders you needed for the care of your client?

Receiving, preparing, and giving accurate and timely SBAR reports takes practice. Use every opportunity you have in clinical to give an SBAR report to your clinical instructor, your nurse, or with your instructor's assistance, an SBAR report to a healthcare provider. Each time you give an SBAR report, reflect on what you did well and what could you do next time to improve on your SBAR report. If you are on the receiving end of the SBAR report, ask questions for any information that is missing that you may need.

Please remember to "Repeat back or use the Read back technique" to verify the received information (i.e., orders that include DNR, diagnostic tests, medications, and/or essential components of care, etc.).

SBAR Was Designed to HELP PROMOTE PATIENT SAFETY!

APPENDIX H

EXAMPLE OF SBAR FORMAT TO MAKE
A CALL TO THE HEALTHCARE PROVIDER

Situation:	James Mulhaney 62-year-old male Client of P. Smith, MD Admitted to ED with new onset of erratic behavior at work
Background:	Brought to ED at 1500.

Past Medical History:	Past medical history is only from an employee health fair form the client's coworker brought with them; client is acutely confused and no family has been reached. History of hypertension. Only other known history is a resolved prostate cancer:
	
	Reported medications:
	  Atenolol 25 mg once daily.
	  Oxybutynin chloride 5 mg twice daily.
	  Aspirin 81 mg once daily.

Allergies:	No known drug allergies (NKDA)
Assessment:	He is acutely confused and combative. This is reported to be a new situation today at work that has worsened in the past few hours.
Abnormal assessment findings:	He's oriented to person only, combative and confused statements with some swatting away motions, possible hallucinations Vital signs: Temp–99.6, Heart rate–98 BPM, Respiratory Rate–20/min; Blood Pressure–140/74. His BP on his employee health fair record, from 4 months ago, was higher, 152/80. He has urinated once, 140 ml. His urine is pink-tinged and has a strong odor. He is pale and sweaty. FLACC Pain Score is 5 out of 10. He hasn't received anything for pain.
Code Status:	Unknown
Recommendations:	Initial orders by the ED healthcare provider: • Vital signs and mental status checks hourly. • Regular supervision and safety checks. • Strict I and O. • Regular diet. • Encourage fluids. • Check finger stick blood sugar now. • Consult for an acute psychiatric evaluation

Please remember to "Repeat back or use the Read back technique" to verify the received information (i.e., orders that include DNR, diagnostic tests, medications, and/or essential components of care, etc.).

ENGAGING THE LEARNER ACTIVITIES

STUDENT-CENTERED LEARNING ACTIVITIES
LINKED TO PROFESSIONAL AND NCLEX® STANDARDS

Resources Needed for Activity	*The Eight-Step Approach for Student Clinical Success* (Zager, Manning & Herman, 2018)
Standards	**Student Instructions**
Management of Care Organize workload to manage time effectively.	**Typical Day Schedule Student Guide** (Refer to Appendix B, Typical Day Schedule Student Guide and Appendix C, Typical Day Schedule Student Guide Template) 1. Complete the blank template of the schedule to reflect the requirements of the unit you are assigned. a. Change the schedule as needed each clinical day to reflect your client's needs.

Pharmacological and Parenteral Therapies
 	
Prepare and administer medication, using rights of medication administration.
	Medication Administration Protocol: A Safe Approach
	(Refer to Appendix E)
	
	2. Review the Medication Administration Protocol: A Safe Approach prior to clinical.
	   a. Demonstrate how to follow the Medication Administration Protocol: A Safe Approach.
	   b. Give feedback to your partner.

Management of Care
 	
Provide and receive report on assigned clients.
	SBAR Report
	(Refer to Appendix D, F, and G)
	
	3. Review the components of the SBAR report.
	   a. Prepare a written SBAR report. (Refer to Appendix G)
	   b. Give the SBAR report.
	   c. Use the written client scenario from your instructor or use the examples given in Appendix F and determine what is and is not a priority to report.

Management of Care
 	
Provide and receive report on assigned clients.
	SBAR Report—Missing Information
	(Refer to Appendix D, F, G, and H)
	
	4. Determine what is missing from the SBAR report.
	   a. What additional information is needed if you were giving a report to the next shift?
	   b. What additional information is needed when you are calling the healthcare provider to report a change in client's condition?

NOTES

Improving Clinical Decision Making

IN THIS CHAPTER YOU WILL LEARN HOW TO:

➤ Develop prioritization strategies

➤ Apply inquiry questions

➤ Apply reflection questions

➤ Use thinking strategies to develop clinical decision making

Now that you have a structure for organizing your clinical day, a protocol for medication administration, and a tool to help you organize your care, it is time to help you improve your clinical reasoning skills and ability to prioritize. Critical thinking incorporates the logical realistic judgments that help you clarify what is true and false (Ennis, 1987 in Cannon & Boswell, 2016, p. 18). Clinical reasoning is when you make decisions/judgments about the patient situation. It is the logical process of collecting system-specific assessments, analyzing these, understanding the problem or clinical situation, and planning and implementing interventions (Levett-Jones, 2010). When your clinical instructors ask you questions, they are doing their job! The reason they ask you questions is to understand your thinking and reinforce your learning (Koharchnik, Caputi, Robb, & Culleiton, 2015). Answering questions strengthens your clinical reasoning skills, decision making, your ability to prioritize care, and to evaluate and make judgments about the outcome of the care provided.

DEVELOP PRIORITIZATION STRATEGIES

Prioritization is an expectation of the new graduate, and it is reflected in the type of questions you must answer to be successful on NCLEX®. "This competency requires a new approach to thinking and processing clinical data" (Manning & Zager, 2014, p. 11). What this means to you, is you will need to expand your basic assessments. You will need to compare and contrast your clinical findings to those previously obtained on your client or to your earlier assessment findings.

You need to determine if your assessments are changing over time. Do the assessments indicate the trend is improving or do they indicate a potential complication?

Thinking strategies such as compare, contrast, and trend help you develop your prioritization skills. Prioritizing care to include who to see first, which healthcare provider order to implement first, or what medication should be administered first are great activities to help you gain confidence in your ability to prioritize.

In addition to prioritization, "Today's nurses are expected to know more about interpretation of clinical assessments or laboratory findings than simply the normal and abnormal ranges." (Benner, Sutphen, Leonard, & Day, 2010, p. 27). The next chart compares basic clinical assessments to assessments needed to trend for potential complications using the example of the concept of oxygenation. Review the chart below for questions you need to ask yourself when you are comparing, contrasting, and trending your client's clinical findings.

COMPARISON OF BASIC CLINICAL ASSESSMENTS WITH TRENDING FOR POTENTIAL COMPLICATIONS

BASIC CLINICAL ASSESSMENTS	TREND FOR POTENTIAL COMPLICATIONS
Medical Diagnosis: Chronic Obstructive Pulmonary Disease	System-Specific Pathophysiology: Obstructive airflow that impedes respirations–Concept: Oxygenation (altered)
1. Respiratory Rate?	1. Respiratory Rate? • Compare, contrast, and trend from previous assessment (i.e., shallow, nasal flaring present, etc.). • Has client just received a narcotic that may affect the breathing?
2. Breath sounds? Equality?	2. Breath sounds? Equality? • Compare, contrast, and trend from previous assessment (i.e., adventitious sounds, use of accessory muscles, etc.).
3. O_2 saturation?	3. O_2 saturation? • Is the finger cold? • Is the probe in appropriate place? • Is it connected to monitor? • Does the client have the appropriate amount of oxygen with the correct delivery system (i.e., nasal cannula, mask, etc.)? • Does the client have peripheral vascular insufficiency such as Raynaud's Disease?
4. Hypoxia?	4. Is the client presenting with **early** versus **late** signs of hypoxia? • Early: restless, increase in the HR and RR. • Late: confusion, decrease in the HR and RR.

COMPARISON OF BASIC CLINICAL ASSESSMENTS
WITH TRENDING FOR POTENTIAL COMPLICATIONS *(cont'd)*

BASIC CLINICAL ASSESSMENTS	TREND FOR POTENTIAL COMPLICATIONS
Medical Diagnosis: Chronic Obstructive Pulmonary Disease	System-Specific Pathophysiology: Obstructive airflow that impedes respirations–Concept: Oxygenation (altered)
5. Arterial blood gas values?	5. Arterial blood gas values: • Trending from previous values. • Is the client currently experiencing changes (i.e., RR, breath sounds, shallow respirations, etc.)?
6. Look at the blood gas values of three clients in the right column. Which client should be assessed first?	6. Which of these three clients should be assessed first based on their arterial blood gas values? a. A client with COPD who has RR 18/min and in one hour increased to 24/min. b. A client with COPD with RR 22/min. c. A client with asthma who had an acute exacerbation with audible wheezing 30 minutes ago. Rationale: Prioritization is more than just relying on the "ABC's" for the correct answer. You must make a clinical decision based on the client that requires immediate action. This would make the correct answer client c. Options a and b are chronic with no immediate distress. Option c is an acute problem that mandates immediate assessment and/or intervention. They all have airway complications!
7. Look at the clinical assessment findings of three clients with COPD. Which clinical assessment findings indicates an expected outcome from the nursing care for a client with COPD?	7. Which of these clinical assessment findings indicate an expected outcome from the nursing care for a client with COPD? a. Client presents with clear breath sounds. b. Client presents with an O_2 sat of 94% that increased from 86% three hours ago. c. Client with COPD participates in physical activity with no shortness of breath. Rationale: Option b is the answer and reflects the expected outcome for this client with COPD. Options a and c are unrealistic for this client. In order to answer the question, it is imperative to recognize normal findings for a client with COPD. It is not as easy as using the ABCs! It is imperative to compare and review trends in order to make a clinical decision.

Manning, L & Zager, L. (2014). Medical surgical nursing concepts made insanely easy: A new approach to prioritizing nursing! Duluth, GA: I CAN Publishing, Inc. p. 12.

The "SAFETY" Model (Appendix A) is a systematic approach to help you determine your client's priority needs. How to use the "SAFETY" model in the care of your client is illustrated in Chapter 5 of this book.

SAFETY: A New Systematic Approach to Prioritize Nursing Care Based on Standards (Appendix B) is a tool to assist you as you learn the "SAFETY" Model and the prioritization process. Your clinical reasoning skills will develop as you begin to understand there can be many reasons why a client and/or a situation is a priority besides having airway and circulation issues. The priority could be a safety issue with a client who is at risk for committing suicide or it could be that the nurse needs to intervene because of a standard of practice is not being followed or to question a new order from the healthcare provider. The "SAFETY" model is discussed in detail in Chapter 8 with strategies on how to use it throughout clinical and in the classroom. For additional information on prioritizing concepts, refer to the book *Medical Surgical Nursing Concepts Made Insanely Easy: A New Approach to Prioritizing Nursing!* (Manning & Zager, 2014).

APPLY INQUIRY QUESTIONS

Inquiry questions asked by your clinical instructors require revealing what you know. It is essential to answer questions that take you beyond memorization of facts to apply the information to a specific client and be able to make clinical decisions about the client's care. Answering inquiry questions helps your clinical instructor and you determine if you know how to give safe and effective care (Pesut & Herman, 1999). Inquiry questions also help you learn the kind of questions you need to ask yourself when the clinical instructor is not present.

+ Do I know the basic facts /information about the topic?

+ Can I apply the information to the client's situation?

+ Can I decide among the potential options, what is the best plan of care for my client?

+ How does this client's care compare to other similar clients I have cared for?

+ Can I think of examples where I could apply the same plan of care for future clients?

With more clinical experiences, you will begin to create a pattern of care for a particular type of client. The chart at the top of page 31 provides examples of how inquiry questions can help you develop more advanced clinical reasoning skills.

The Quick Approach: Inquiry Questions for Classroom and Clinical Knowledge Organized Around the "SAFETY" Model (Appendix C) and the "SAFETY" model (Refer to Chapter 8) will provide multiple examples of questions that can be applied in different client care situations. The questions have been written within the framework of the NCLEX-RN® activities that are based on practice and safety standards. You can use these questions as you prepare for clinical and for classroom exams. This is a success formula for the NCLEX-RN®!

Types of Inquiry Questions

DEFINITIONS	EXAMPLES OF INQUIRY QUESTIONS
Knowledge: Memorized information/facts.	What is the normal range for blood pressure?
Application: Connecting knowledge to a clinical situation.	Which is the most important vital sign to monitor in your client who has hypertension?
Analysis: Understanding pros and cons, strengths and weaknesses or other options in decision making.	Should you administer the antihypertensive medication as ordered for a client who has a blood pressure of 95/60?
Synthesis: Pulling together multiple sources of experiences, data and information to make decisions about needed client care. This process may require asking yourself several inquiry questions.	What has the blood pressure been for the past two days? Is this the same or has there been a change? What could be contributing to the change in the BP? Are there any guidelines in the healthcare provider's orders regarding their BP? What are the priority nursing actions?

APPLY REFLECTION QUESTIONS

Reflection questions require you to think about your own thinking. Reflection challenges you to self-monitor, plan, and revise your own thinking so you can quickly self-correct (Pesut & Herman, 1999). **Example of Reflection Questions** (Appendix D) can be used to reflect on your clinical experience for the day. You may be asked to share your reflections in a post conference. This example includes points that are a part of the **Rubric for the Concept Map** (Chapter 4, Appendix B). Reflective thinking is an essential component of clinical reasoning (Koharchnik, Caputi, Robb, & Culleiton, 2015).

The **Urinary Catheterization Algorithm** (Appendix E) illustrates how your clinical instructor might use inquiry and reflection questions before, during, and after a urinary catheterization. The questions included in the algorithm help you see beyond the task to the clinical decision making and judgment needed even with procedures. These same types of questions apply to any procedure. Use the **Procedure Algorithm Template** (Appendix F) for any procedure or task you are doing in clinical. This will help you prepare and to think beyond the procedure to provide quality care and to intervene early to prevent potential complications.

USE THINKING STRATEGIES FOR CLINICAL DECISION MAKING

Clinical decision making is a skill that can be learned. **Thinking Strategies to Improve Student's Clinical Decision Making** (Appendix G), lists thinking strategies, their definitions, and how to use them in clinical. The chart combines thinking strategies with inquiry and reflection questions. If you use the thinking strategies in the chart, you will improve your clinical reasoning.

APPENDIX A

"SAFETY" MODEL
The following describes the components of the "SAFETY" Model.
THE "SAFETY" MODEL FOR CLASSROOM, CLINICAL AND TESTING

S   **S**ystem-Specific Pathophysiology, Assessments, Labs and Diagnostic Procedures

A   **A**nalysis of Concepts

F   **F**irst-Do Priority Nursing Interventions
      First-Do Medications

E   **E**valuation of Expected Outcomes

T   **T**rend For Potential Complications

Y   **Y**ou Must Manage Care to Prevent **"RISK"** to the Client

The **S** in **"SAFETY"** represents **System-Specific Pathophysiology** and **System-Specific Assessments**. **System-Specific Pathophysiology** organizes diseases around the pathophysiology for a specific system. The key to linking concepts to other diseases is to understand the physiological changes that are occurring with the client; you must know the "why"! **System-Specific Assessments** are discussed with a focus on pathophysiology. The process of being able to not only know the assessments but be able to recognize early versus late clinical findings is a journey! Reviewing and analyzing labs and diagnostic procedures findings will assist you to connect the significance of these to your client. The good news is you will quickly recognize, for example, 15 diseases involving the respiratory system will result in the same system-specific assessment findings for the concept of oxygenation.

The **A** in **"SAFETY"** stands for **Analyzing Priority Concepts**. Once the assessments have been completed and reviewed analyze the system-specific assessment to determine the priority concept(s). Knowing the concept will help you prioritize the care required for this client.

The **F** in **"SAFETY"** represents **First-Do Priority Interventions**. The interventions represent the priority interventions for that specific concept. However, the interventions are not in order of priority because they depend on the clinical situation. The interventions also include medications (refer to the book *Pharmacology Made Insanely Easy*).

The **E** in **"SAFETY"** represents **Evaluation of Expected Outcomes** from nursing care as well as from the administration of medications. The evaluation of outcomes will represent the return of clinical assessments within the defined limits (WDL) (refer to the book *Medical Surgical Nursing Concepts Made Insanely Easy!*).

The **T** in **"SAFETY"** is **TREND for Potential Complications**. A very important component of clinical judgment is to be competent in comparing, contrasting, and trending ongoing system assessments, lab results, and/ or changes in the client's condition that require intervention. This is a skill that has to be developed over time. It begins with knowing the normal clinical findings specific to the concept and progressing to the ability to differentiate between early and late clinical findings.

The **Y** in **"SAFETY"** stands for **You Must Manage Care to Prevent "RISK" to the Client**. The mnemonic **"RISK"** is a valuable tool to organize and reflect the priority-management standards.

R   **R**oom Assignments, **R**ecognize limitations of staff, **R**estraint safety, **R**isk for falls, **R**eceive or give report

I   **I**dentify trends, **I**nfection control, **I**dentification of client, **I**dentify accuracy of orders, **I**nformed consent, **I**nterdisciplinary Team Collaboration

S   **S**kin breakdown, **S**afe equipment, **S**cope of Practice for delegation

K   **K**now Standards of Practice, **K**now how to document, **K**now how to prepare for transfer, discharge, **K**now how to teach and incorporate health-promotion activities

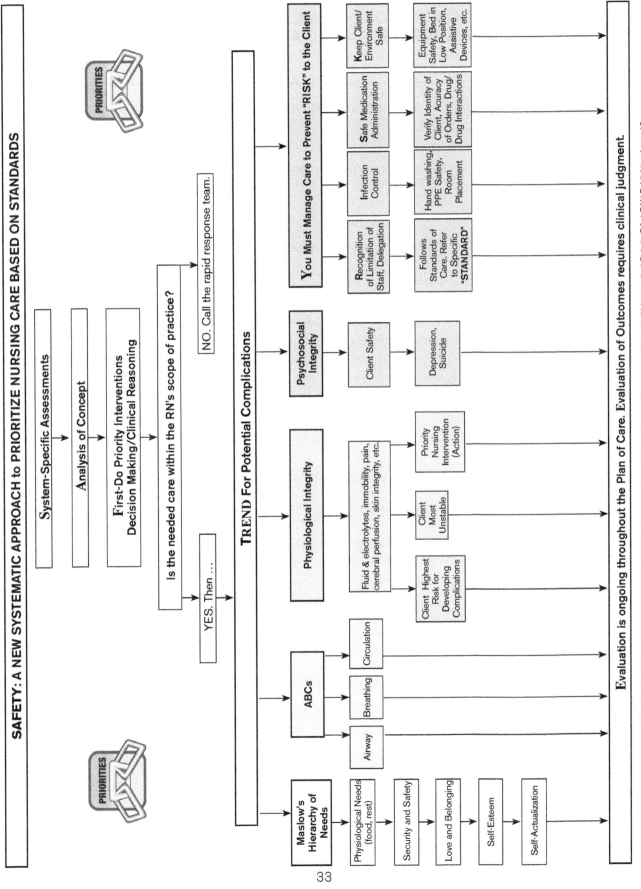

SAFETY: A NEW SYSTEMATIC APPROACH to PRIORITIZE NURSING CARE BASED ON STANDARDS

PRIORITIES

System-Specific Assessments

Analysis of Concept

First-Do Priority Interventions
Decision Making/Clinical Reasoning

Is the needed care within the RN's scope of practice?

NO. Call the rapid response team.

YES. Then ....

TREND For Potential Complications

Maslow's Hierarchy of Needs
- Physiological Needs (food, rest)
- Security and Safety
- Love and Belonging
- Self-Esteem
- Self-Actualization

ABCs
- Airway
- Breathing
- Circulation

Physiological Integrity
- Client Highest Risk for Developing Complications
- Client Most Unstable
- Fluid & electrolytes, immobility, pain, cerebral perfusion, skin integrity, etc.
- Priority Nursing Intervention (Action)

Psychosocial Integrity
- Client Safety
- Depression, Suicide

You Must Manage Care to Prevent "RISK" to the Client
- Recognition of Limitation of Staff, Delegation
  - Follows Standards of Care. Refer to Specific "STANDARD"
- Infection Control
  - Hand washing, PPE Safety, Room Placement
- Safe Medication Administration
  - Verify Identity of Client, Accuracy of Orders, Drug/ Drug Interactions
- Keep Client/ Environment Safe
  - Equipment Safety, Bed in Low Position, Assistive Devices, etc.

PRIORITIES

Evaluation is ongoing throughout the Plan of Care. Evaluation of Outcomes requires clinical judgment.

Manning, L. and Zager, L. © 2014 Medical surgical nursing concepts made insanely easy: A new approach to prioritizing nursing! Duluth, GA: I CAN Publishing, Inc. p.13.

33

APPENDIX C

THE QUICK APPROACH: INQUIRY QUESTIONS FOR CLASSROOM AND CLINICAL KNOWLEDGE ORGANIZED AROUND THE "SAFETY" MODEL
(Adapted from the 2018 RN Practice Analysis)

SYSTEM-SPECIFIC PATHOPHYSIOLOGY

1. Which of these clinical assessment findings indicate a complication with the pathophysiology related to a **Specific Disease** (acute or chronic)?

2. Which of these statements made by **the nurse, client, or family** indicates an understanding of the pathophysiology for a client diagnosed with a **Specific Disease** (acute or chronic)?

SYSTEM-SPECIFIC ASSESSMENTS

1. Which vital sign assessments would be the highest priority for a client with a specific diagnosis (i.e., temperature, pulse, respiratory rate, and blood pressure) and why?

2. Which of these vital signs should be reported to a team member or provider of care for a client who is one hour post-op for a **tonsillectomy (specific diagnosis or procedure)**?

3. Which assessments would be a priority for your client (i.e., BP, bradycardia, bleeding, etc.) and why?

4. Which assessment finding is a priority for monitoring your client's hydration status (i.e., I & O, edema, signs and symptoms of dehydration)?

5. Which of your clients should be assessed/triaged initially and why?

6. Which focused assessment (or system-specific assessment) would require immediate intervention following shift report?

7. Which focused assessment (or system-specific assessment) for a client with a **specific diagnosis** would require further intervention?

8. Which systems-specific assessment or reassessments would be the priority for your client and why (**i.e., GI, respiratory, cardiac, etc.**)?

9. Which steps would be most appropriate when performing a focused assessment for (i.e., gastrointestinal, respiratory, cardiac)?

10. Which of the psychosocial, spiritual, cultural and occupational assessment findings may affect the client's care (i.e., cultural—dietary, occupational—stress, etc.)?

11. What assessments are important for planning your client's care during hospitalization (i.e., food, latex, and environmental allergies)?

12. What is important to assess with your client when learning new information about a stressful treatment plan (non-verbal cues from the psychological or physical stressor)?

13. Which assessment findings indicate an older client understands how to or has the ability to manage self-care in the home environment (i.e., community resources)?

SYSTEM-SPECIFIC LABS/TESTS

1. Place options in chronological order when obtaining a **specific diagnostic test** (i.e., glucometer).

2. Which of these clinical findings would be a priority to report for a client who is post **the test** (i.e., **lab test, biopsy, cardiac cath, etc.**)?

3. Which of these clinical assessment findings would require immediate intervention to prevent a complication for a client who is experiencing **the procedure**?

4. Which of these clinical assessment findings from a **specific diagnostic test** would require further intervention?

THE QUICK APPROACH: INQUIRY QUESTIONS FOR CLASSROOM AND CLINICAL KNOWLEDGE ORGANIZED AROUND THE "SAFETY" MODEL *(cont'd)*

ANALYSIS & CONNECTED PRIORITY NURSING CONCEPT

1. Based on the information received in shift report, which client would require an immediate nursing intervention?

2. Which client should be assessed first in order to assist with time management?

3. Which signs and symptoms indicate a complication from *a specific drug, medical condition, etc.*?

4. Place in order of care delivery how you would assess/triage these four clients.

5. Which of these clinical findings indicates a change in client's condition and needs immediate intervention?

6. Which client would be a priority for the nurse to assess first following shift report?

7. Which of these changes in the client's condition requires immediate intervention?

FIRST-DO PLANS AND INTERVENTIONS

Plans

1. Which plan would be most effective for maintaining client confidentiality/privacy?

2. What plan would be most important for a client with *Diabetes Insipidus* (*or any condition that requires calculation of the I & O for client*)?

3. Which behavioral management techniques would be most useful in the plan for a client who is presenting with *a specific disorder* (i.e., manipulative)?

4. What plan would be highest priority for assisting a client to sleep/rest after being discharged from the hospital?

5. What plan would be the highest priority for a client with an alteration in nutritional intake (*i.e., anorexia, pica, anemia, gastroenteritis, colitis, etc.*) (i.e., adjust diet, monitor height and weight, include food preferences, etc.)?

6. What plan would be important to include when teaching a client/family member(s) about a procedure/treatment/medical condition/medication, etc. ?

Interventions

1. What is the priority nursing action for a client with a *fluid and electrolyte imbalance (specific concept, i.e., hypo/hypercalcemia, hypo/hyperkalemia, increase in intracranial pressure, hypothermia, etc.)*?

2. What is the priority nursing intervention for a client with a *sodium level of 128 mEq*/or *any alteration in a lab value* (i.e., serum glucose, serum potassium, etc.)?

3. What nursing intervention has the highest priority for promoting infection control for a client with a *specific disease/organism* (i.e., TB, Rubella, Clostridium difficile, Hepatitis A, etc.)?

4. When communicating with your client, what is your best response?

5. What therapeutic communication techniques were used to support your client or family and/or increase client understanding of his/her behavior?

6. What intervention(s) would be effective in assisting client with emotional and spiritual needs?

7. Which intervention(s) would be the highest priority to manage/prevent possible complications of your client's condition and/or procedure (i.e., circulatory complications, seizures, aspiration, potential neurological complications, etc.) or a client on a ventilator?

8. What would be the priority of care for a client who has been physically abused? (advocate, report, etc.)

9. What intervention was used to provide client and family with information about condition/illness, expected progression, and/or possible outcomes?

cont'd on next page

THE QUICK APPROACH: INQUIRY QUESTIONS FOR CLASSROOM AND CLINICAL KNOWLEDGE ORGANIZED AROUND THE "SAFETY" MODEL *(cont'd)*

10. What procedures did you implement in order to admit, transfer, or discharge the client?

11. What steps did you take in discontinuing or removing: IV, NG, urethral catheter, or other lines or tubes?

12. Which nursing intervention would be a priority for providing therapy for comfort and treatment of inflammation, swelling (i.e., apply heat and cold treatments, elevate limb, etc.)?

13. What are the appropriate steps in performing or assisting with a dressing change (i.e., wound, central line dressing, etc.)?

14. How can you provide the appropriate support to a client coping with life changes?

15. What is the priority of care when transcribing healthcare provider orders for a new prescription for $MgSO_4$? *(Unapproved abbreviation)*

16. Which nursing action is appropriate for proper lifting, assistive devices, etc. *(using ergonomic principles)*?

17. What nursing action would be appropriate for a client with a new order that you have limited knowledge about (i.e., *information technology such as computer, video, etc.*)?

18. What nursing action is the highest priority for handling bio-hazardous materials?

19. Which nursing action is highest priority when inserting, maintaining, or removing a peripheral intravenous line?

20. When managing the client on telemetry, which assessment finding should be reported for a client with a suspected **myocardial infarction or any condition that would alter the cardiac rhythm** (i.e., angina, hyperkalemia, hypokalemia, overdose of digitalis, etc.)?

21. Which intervention is the highest priority for a client with an alteration in **elimination** (i.e., **cystitis, constipation, diarrhea, etc.**)?

22. When providing care what evidence-based practice/research results did you use for providing quality care to your client?

23. What nursing action is the highest priority immediately prior to the client going to **specific surgery or procedure** in the AM? *(Answer: Check that informed consent is on the chart.)*

24. What nursing action is the highest priority immediately 2 days prior to the client going to **specific surgery or procedure**? *(Answer: Verify client comprehends and consents to care/procedures, including procedures requiring informed consent.)*

25. What nursing care would be most appropriate for a client with (i.e., **anxiety, depression, dementia, eating disorders**)?

26. What is the priority of care for a client presenting with **specific clinical findings** indicating alteration in hemodynamics tissue perfusion and hemostasis (i.e., cerebral, cardiac, peripheral)?

27. What nursing care is a priority following a **specific surgery** and is presenting with **specific clinical assessment findings** (i.e., thyroidectomy, tonsillectomy, GI surgery, hysterectomy, etc.)?

FIRST-DO MEDICATIONS

1. Prior to administering the medication, which data would be most pertinent to review (i.e., vital signs, lab results, allergies, etc.)?

2. When adjusting or titrating dosage of medications, what physiological parameters did you use (i.e., giving insulin according to blood sugar levels, titrating medication to maintain a specified blood pressure, etc.)?

3. Which nursing actions will be most appropriate with medication administration (using the rights of medication administration)?

THE QUICK APPROACH: INQUIRY QUESTIONS FOR CLASSROOM AND CLINICAL KNOWLEDGE ORGANIZED AROUND THE "SAFETY" MODEL *(cont'd)*

4. During an IV infusion, what is most important to monitor and maintain (*i.e., infusion site, equipment, flushing infusion devices, checking, rates, fluid, and sites, etc.*)?

5. What is the priority intervention for your client who is receiving medication by the *intravenous route* (*i.e., IVP, IVPB, PCA pump, continuous infusion fluids, parenteral nutrition) or by SC, IM, intradermal or topical or in the form of eye, ear or nose drops, sprays, ointments or by inhalation (including nebulizer or metered dose inhaler*)?

6. Which calculations did you use for medication administration?

7. What regulations did you comply with when working with controlled substances (i.e., counting narcotics, wasting narcotics, etc.)?

8. What information did you share with the client/family regarding the medication regimen, treatments, and/or procedures?

9. What would be the priority of care when transcribing healthcare provider orders for a new prescription for **MgSO$_4$**?

10. What steps are most important when administering medications by the oral route or gastric tube (i.e., po, sublingual, nasogastric tube, G tube, etc.)?

11. What plan is most appropriate for preparing medication for administration (i.e., crush medications as needed and appropriate, place in appropriate administrative device, assemble equipment, etc.)?

12. What should be included in the plan to avoid when administering medications (i.e., food, fluids, and other drugs) to minimize medication interactions?

13. What clinical outcomes best determine the effect of the (*pain medication—specific medication*)?

14. What clinical findings are expected when the dopamine dosage is titrated appropriately?

15. What clinical findings are expected when the insulin is titrated according to the blood sugar levels?

16. Which assessment findings indicate a positive outcome from the albuterol (Ventolin) treatment?

17. Which assessment findings indicate positive outcomes from (*specific medications*)?

18. Which documentation indicates the nurse understands standard terminology and how to use approved abbreviations?

19. Which clinical findings indicate a therapeutic effect from **a specific drug**?

20. What is most important to monitor for a client with (i.e., central, PICC, epidural, and venous access)?

21. What plan for a client taking **warfarin (Coumadin)** (**or a specific medication**) would reflect care within the legal scope of practice?

22. What is the priority of care for a client prior to the nurse initiating any procedure, care, or medication administration?

23. What information is most important to include in the teaching plan for a client who has an order for (*specific medication*)?

24. What is the priority of care for a client who has a central line?

25. Which of these **medications** should the nurse question the appropriateness for a specific client?

26. Which of these **orders** should the nurse question?

27. Which of these **orders** should be verified for appropriateness/accuracy?

28. What would be the priority of care for a LPN who administered (*specific medication such as propranolol*) for a client with asthma?

cont'd on next page

APPENDIX C

THE QUICK APPROACH: INQUIRY QUESTIONS FOR CLASSROOM AND CLINICAL KNOWLEDGE ORGANIZED AROUND THE "SAFETY" MODEL *(cont'd)*

29. Which of these assessment findings require immediate intervention?

30. Which plan is priority for a client when the nurse is administering medication in order to maintain a safe and controlled environment?

PROCEDURES

1. After a specific diagnostic test (*i.e., **cardiac catheterization, liver biopsy, stress test, etc.***), what clinical outcomes indicate a complication?

2. Which of these results from (***a specific diagnostic test***) indicate a complication?

3. When performing a diagnostic test (i.e., O_2 saturation, glucose monitoring, testing for occult blood, gastric pH, urine specific gravity, etc.) what are the most important interventions?

4. What nursing action would be important for the nurse to implement prior to performing a specific diagnostic test? (i.e., electrocardiogram, oxygen saturation, glucose monitoring, etc.)

5. What nursing intervention would be highest priority for a client who has (***a specific complication after a diagnostic test***) (*i.e., bleeding after a liver biopsy, bleeding after a cardiac catheterization, etc.*)

6. What nursing action would be important when obtaining ***a urine specimen from a catheter*** or (*i.e., wound specimen, stool, etc.*)?

7. Which information would be important to teach a client regarding ***a specific treatment/procedure***?

8. Which clinical findings following a (***specific diagnostic test***) require further intervention in order to prevent complications?

9. What is important to include in the plan when assisting with an invasive procedure (*i.e., **thoracentesis, bronchoscopy, etc.***)?

10. Which of these vital signs following a (***specific diagnostic test***) require further intervention?

EVALUATION OF EXPECTED OUTCOMES

1. What clinical findings indicate effectiveness of treatment for a client with ***a specific acute or chronic diagnosis***? (*i.e., Parkinson's Disease, Multiple Sclerosis, etc.*)

2. What is important to evaluate with the client who is using a device to promote venous return such as (*i.e., anti-embolic stockings, sequential compression devices*)?

3. What plan would be appropriate for evaluating the care of a client (*i.e., **evaluate care map, clinical pathway, etc.***)?

4. What documentation is most appropriate for a procedure, treatment, or medication and what is the client's response?

5. Is the medication order appropriate for your client (*i.e., **appropriate for the client's condition, given by appropriate route, in appropriate dosage, etc.***)?

6. What documentation in the chart indicates an understanding of the appropriate education necessary for client and family regarding pain management?

7. Which documentation evaluates teaching performed and the level of understanding of client, family or staff?

8. Which documentation indicates the client and family have been educated about his/her rights and responsibilities?

9. Which documentation indicates that the client has given informed consent for treatment?

10. What assessment findings indicate an improvement in the client's hydration status?

THE QUICK APPROACH: INQUIRY QUESTIONS FOR CLASSROOM AND CLINICAL KNOWLEDGE ORGANIZED AROUND THE "SAFETY" MODEL *(cont'd)*

11. After initiating the plan of care, how did you evaluate the client care (i.e., multidisciplinary care plan, care map, critical pathway, etc.)?

12. Which clinical findings indicate a need to evaluate the client's weight?

13. What clinical outcomes best determine the effect of the pain medication?

14. What assessment findings indicate an improvement in the client's hydration status?

15. What clinical assessment findings indicate desired outcomes from a (*i.e., specific medication, intervention, procedure, test, etc.*)?

16. What clinical assessment findings indicate a complication from a (*i.e., specific medication, intervention, procedure, test, etc.*)?

TREND POTENTIAL COMPLICATIONS

1. Which trends and changes in client condition require further intervention?

2. Which signs and symptoms indicate complications? What is the priority intervention?

3. Which vital signs, I & O, hemodynamic readings, intracranial pressure readings, Glasgow Coma Scale number, lab values, breath sounds, etc. require further evaluation and intervention?

YOU MUST MANAGE CARE: PREVENT "RISKS"

Room Assignments, **R**ecognize limitations of staff, **R**estraint safety, **R**isk for falls, **R**ecognize cost-effective care

1. Which plan would be most appropriate to protect your client from injury (*i.e., falls, electrical hazards, malfunctioning equipment, rugs, clutter, etc.*)?

2. What is the plan for assisting the client in the performance of activities of daily living (*i.e., ambulation, reposition, hygiene, transfer to chair, eating, toileting, etc.*)?

3. What plan is most important to develop after evaluating the risk assessment profile for your client (*i.e., sensory impairment, potential for falls, level of mobility, etc.*) *and why*?

4. What plan would be most cost-effective for the nurse manager to implement on medical surgical unit?

5. Which of the clients would be most appropriate to transfer to the (i.e., medical surgical unit, orthopedic, psychiatric, etc.) unit?

6. While supervising the (i.e., UAP, LPN, RN) the nurse observes the **UAP (palpating the abdomen of a child with Wilm's tumor)** (*include an unsafe nursing practice*). What would be the priority nursing action?

7. What would be the priority action from the charge nurse for a LPN who administered **propranolol or a specific medication** for a client with **asthma or a specific disease**?

8. What room assignment would be most appropriate for a client with TB?

9. What is the priority of care for a client with an order for restraints?

10. Which nursing action for a client with restraints on requires immediate intervention?

cont'd on next page

APPENDIX C

THE QUICK APPROACH: INQUIRY QUESTIONS FOR CLASSROOM AND CLINICAL KNOWLEDGE ORGANIZED AROUND THE "SAFETY" MODEL *(cont'd)*

Infection Control, **I**dentification of client, **I**dentify accuracy of orders, **I**nformed consent, **I**nterdisciplinary Collaboration

1. Which **assessment findings** would result in the nurse developing a plan to collaborate with *other disciplines* (i.e., physician, RT, PT, radiology, dietary, lab, etc.) while providing care to the client with a **specific diagnosis**?

2. What would be a priority plan for a client who is providing care for husband with (*i.e., Alzheimer's Disease—or a specific disease*) and is presenting with (*i.e., fatigue and weight loss—or specific assessment findings*)? (*referral*)

3. What nursing intervention would have the highest priority for promoting infection control for a client with **the specific communicable disease (i.e., TB, C. Diff, Salmonella, etc.)**?

4. Which nursing actions indicate an understanding of safe care for a client with **tuberculosis (specific disease)**?

5. What would be the priority of care when transcribing the healthcare provider's new order for a prescription for **MgSO$_4$**?

6. What is the priority of care for a client presenting with delusions who needs a medication and does not have an arm bracelet on for identification?

7. What is the priority of care for a client prior to going to surgery?

Skin breakdown, **S**afe equipment, **S**tandard of Practice, **S**cope of Practice for delegation

1. What is the priority plan for maintaining your client's skin integrity (i.e., skin care, turn client, etc.)?

2. What plan is most appropriate when using equipment in performing **specific client care procedures and treatment**?

3. What is the appropriate nursing care for **devices and equipment** used for drainage (i.e., surgical wound drains, chest tube suction, or drainage devices, urethral catheter care, etc.)?

4. Which **level of nursing personnel** would be most appropriate to assign to a client with **specific condition/assessments**, etc. when making out assignments (i.e., LPN, VN, assistive personnel, other RNs, etc.)?

5. Which of these nursing interventions are consistent with the Standards of Practice for a client with a **specific disease**?

Know how to Document, **K**now how to Teach, **K**now Ethical Practice, **K**now Growth and Development

1. Which plan would be most important in meeting the special needs of the adult client who is (**? years old**) (19-64 years of age)?

2. Which plan would be most important in meeting the special needs of the adult client who is (**? years old**) (65-85 years of age) (over 85 years)?

3. What would be a plan necessary for the parents of a newborn (*i.e., education*)?

4. What information regarding healthy behaviors and health promotion / maintenance recommendations would be appropriate for (*i.e., pregnant woman, infant, post-menopausal, smoker, etc.*)?

5. What is important to include in the discharge teaching plan for a client going home after being diagnosed with a **cerebral vascular accident** (*i.e., home safety issues*)?

6. What nursing action indicates the nurse understands the code of ethics for the registered nurse?

7. Which documentation indicates client understands newly learned information?

8. Which documentation indicates an understanding of safe medication administration for a client who received (*i.e. specific medication*)?

Adapted from NCSBN, 2018. *Organized within the SAFETY Model* by I CAN Publishing, Inc., 2018

EXAMPLE OF REFLECTION QUESTIONS

Student Name _____ Clinical Instructor _____

Sec # _____ Date_____ Sat/UnSat or Grade_____

Date due to Clinical Instructor: _____

Six (6) points are possible and will be added to Rubric Grading Tool for the Concept Map (see Chapter 4, Appendix B)

1. Connect the clinical findings (diagnostic test results) to the priority interventions (medications, treatments) for your client and provide the rationale. (2 points)

2. Based on your analysis of the concepts, what are the expected outcomes for your client? (2 points)

3. What went well today for you in clinical and why? (1 point)

4. What would you do differently if you could and why? (1 point)

APPENDIX E

URINARY CATHETERIZATION ALGORITHM

Expected Outcome: Urinary flow established through the catheter while maintaining asepsis and client comfort.

Inquiry and Reflection Questions about Insertion of a Foley Catheter

Why does this client need a Foley catheter? (Application)

Possible answers: Fluid management, incontinence, post-op renal or urinary procedures

What are potential complications for this client with a Foley catheter? (Application)

Possible answers: Urinary tract infections, skin irritations

What is important to assess in this client with a Foley catheter? (Application)

Possible answers: I & O, signs of infection, color, odor, amount of urine

What are the infection control issues for this client with a Foley catheter? (Application)

Possible answers: Sterile procedure, potential UTI from the catheter, obtaining specimens

Have you done this procedure before?

YES   NO

What went well with the procedure? (Assessing)   Name steps of procedure. (Knowledge)
Did the procedure go as planned? (Reflection)   What potential complications do you anticipate
What will you do differently next time? (Reflection)   with this client? (Analysis)
                                                         What are possible solutions to these
                                                             potential complications? (Analysis)

Clinical instructor observes you doing the procedure.

Clinical instructor evaluates the procedure or process.

Were you able to give individualized care with the task?

T –   Techniques of communication with consideration of the individual

A –   Assessment, A & P, Asepsis

S –   Safety

K –   Knowledge and correct implementation of the procedure/skill

YES   NO

Receive positive feedback based on **TASK**.   Receive feedback on specific areas for improvement.

Evaluation form reflects performance.   Evaluation form reflects performance and areas
                                                          for improvement before performing the procedure
                                                          again.

PROCEDURE ALGORITHM TEMPLATE

Expected outcome for the procedure you are doing: _____

Inquiry and Reflection Questions about the procedure:

Why does this client need _____? (Application)

    Possible answers: _____

What are potential complications from the procedure for this client? (Application)

    Possible answers: _____

What is important to assess in this client? (Application)

    Possible answers: _____

What are the infection control issues for this client? (Application)

    Possible answers: _____

Have you done this procedure before?

YES   NO

What went well with the procedure? (Assessing)
Did the procedure go as planned? (Reflection)
What will you do differently next time? (Reflection)

Name steps of procedure. (Knowledge)
What potential complications do you anticipate
   with this client? (Analysis)
What are possible solutions to these
   potential complications? (Analysis)

Clinical instructor observes you doing the procedure.

Clinical instructor evaluates the procedure or process.

Were you able to give individualized care with the task?

T – Techniques of communication with consideration of the individual

A – Assessment, A & P, Asepsis

S – Safety

K – Knowledge and correct implementation of the procedure/skill

YES   NO

Receive positive feedback based on **TASK**.

Evaluation form reflects performance.

Receive feedback on specific areas for improvement.

Evaluation form reflects performance and areas
   for improvement before performing the procedure
   again

APPENDIX G

Chapter 3

THINKING STRATEGIES TO IMPROVE STUDENTS' CLINICAL DECISION MAKING

Thinking Strategies	Definitions	Inquiry Question Examples	Reflection Question Examples
Knowledge Work	• Active use of reading, memorizing, drilling, writing, reviewing, and practicing to learn clinical vocabulary and facts.	• Why does a client with heart failure have edema?	• What knowledge did I need about heart failure that I did not know? • What do I need to know before I care for a heart failure client again?
Prototype Identification	• Using a model case as a reference point for comparing and contrasting the clinical findings of your client.	• How would a prototype case of heart failure present?	• Were you able to recognize how your client was different from the prototype? • What changes will you make in the care you give next time?
Hypothesizing	• Generating potential concepts based on the pathophysiology of the medical condition. • Recognizing multiple approaches to an outcome or problem.	• What system-specific assess-ments do you need to confirm or change your analysis of your concepts? • Based on your confirmed analysis of the concepts, what are your priority interventions (plan of care)?	• Was I able to identify the appropriate concepts and interventions for my client? • If not, what could I do differently?
Self-Talk	• Expressing one's thoughts to one's self.	• Talk aloud to me about how you will auscultate your client's lung sounds.	• Was I able to auscultate the lung sounds correctly; and if so, do I need to change my priority interventions?
Schema Search	• Accessing general/specific patterns of past experiences that might apply to the current case.	• How does this heart failure client compare to the heart failure client you took care of last week?	• Based on my experiences with heart failure clients, what patterns of care do I see?

THINKING STRATEGIES TO IMPROVE STUDENTS'
CLINICAL DECISION MAKING *(cont'd)*

Thinking Strategies	Definitions	Inquiry Question Examples	Reflection Question Examples
If–Then Thinking	• Connecting ideas and consequences together in a logical sequence.	• If you give the medication now, what will happen? If you hold the medication, what will happen?	• Did I make the right decision about giving/ holding the medication? If not, what would I do differently next time?
Compare & Contrast	• Comparing the strengths and weaknesses of competing alternatives.	• What would be the most effective priority intervention(s) to help improve this client's breathing?	• Did I choose the most effective intervention to improve my client's breathing? • How did I know the intervention was effective?
Trending	• Comparing the client's clinical presentation from one observation to the next observation during the clinical day.	• What were the trends you identified in the assessments you made of your client? • Are there any changes in your assessment? • What actions do you need to take based on your assessment?	• Was I able to identify the trends and changes accurately? • Were your actions appropriate? • If yes, I knew because … • If no, I would do what differently?

ENGAGING THE LEARNER ACTIVITIES

STUDENT-CENTERED LEARNING ACTIVITIES
LINKED TO PROFESSIONAL AND NCLEX® STANDARDS

Resources Needed for Activity	*The Eight-Step Approach for Student Clinical Success* (Zager, Manning & Herman, 2018)
Standards	**Student Instructions**
Physiological integrity; Reduction of Risk Recognize trends and changes in VS, client condition and intervene appropriately; Recognize and prevent signs and symptoms of complications and intervene appropriately.	**Clinical Decision Making Strategies** (Refer to Appendix G, Thinking Strategies to Develop Clinical Decision Making) 1. Based on your clinical day: a. Give an example of how you used "If–Then Thinking" in your clinical decision making. b. Give an example of how you used "Compare and Contrast" for your clinical decision making. c. Give an example how you used "Trending" for your clinical decision making.
Physiological integrity; Reduction of Risk Educate and evaluate accuracy of a treatment order and response to procedures and treatments; Verify appropriateness of an order.	**Clinical Decision Making: Procedures** (Refer to Appendix E, Urinary Catheterization Algorithm and Appendix F, Procedure Template) 2. Work in pairs and answer the questions on the Procedure Template (Appendix F). a. Report your answers to the group. b. Are there similarities in your fellow students answers about their procedures and yours? c. What are the differences? d. How can you apply these questions to other procedures?

The Concept Map

IN THIS CHAPTER YOU WILL LEARN HOW TO:

➤ Create and use a concept map
- ◊ Step 1– Begin with the admitting diagnosis
- ◊ Step 2 – Generate (hypothesize) possible concepts
- ◊ Step 3 – Determine relationships among the concepts
- ◊ Step 4 – Add system-specific assessment findings
- ◊ Step 5 – Determine expected outcomes and outcome/evaluation criteria
- ◊ Step 6 – Determine the priority interventions
- ◊ Step 7 – Evaluate and make clinical judgments about the plan of care
- ◊ Step 8 – Document the care given and client response

➤ Put the concept map into clinical practice

The concept map provides an excellent tool for you to develop your clinical reasoning skills (Daley, Morgan, & Black, 2016). It is a strategy to promote understanding of interrelationships of the client situation and assists you to visualize your plan of care. When your concept map is completed, your clinical instructor can see your thinking to help you improve your clinical decision making skills. We will guide you on a step-by-step approach to creating and using the concept map. The concept map can seem overwhelming when you first look at it, but when you approach it sequentially, it is easy to master.

HOW TO CONSTRUCT AND USE A CONCEPT MAP

When you begin clinical, you will be assigned a client and be given their medical diagnoses. The "SAFETY" Model (see Chapter 8) and the nursing process guide the steps in the development of the concept map.

STEP 1: Begin with the Admitting Diagnoses

Place the admitting medical diagnoses/client situation in the middle of the paper with any client history that would impact the current admission.

Med DX: i.e., heart failure (HF)

Pertinent history/information (i.e., history of chronic renal disease & non-compliance with low-sodium diet, etc.)

Client Age: _____

HT____WT____

Allergies:_____

STEP 2: Generate (Hypothesize) Possible Concepts

Generate (hypothesize) the possible concepts that are pathophysiologically associated with the medical diagnosis(es). Draw a line from the middle circle to each of the hypothesized concepts.

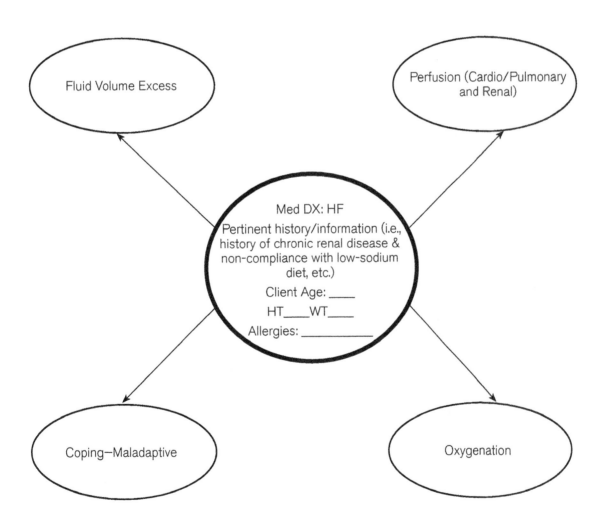

STEP 3: Determine Relationships Among the Concepts

Here is what you would say to yourself to help determine the relationships among the concepts: *"Is there any pathophysiological reason why these two concepts might be related to each other?"* (Refer to Manning & Zager, 2014).

a. *"Is there any pathophysiological reason why perfusion would be related to excess fluid volume?"*

b. In this example, the answer is yes, so draw a line connecting the two concepts.

c. Working systematically around the concept map, you will ask yourself, *"Is perfusion related to the other concepts included on the map?"*

d. Now ask, *"Is there any pathophysiological reason why perfusion is related to oxygenation?"*

e. The answer is yes. Draw a line between the two concepts.

f. Next question, *"Is there any pathophysiological reason why excess fluid volume is related to oxygenation?"*

g. The answer is yes. Draw a line between the two concepts.

h. Next, *"Is there any pathophysiological or logical reason why maladaptive coping is related to fluid volume excess?"*

i. The answer is yes. Draw a line between the two concepts.

j. Finally, *"Is there any pathophysiological reason why maladaptive coping is related to perfusion and/or oxygenation?"*

k. The answer is yes. Both perfusion and oxygenation are indirectly impacted by maladaptive coping (i.e., failure to follow a low-sodium diet) that contributes to fluid volume excess.

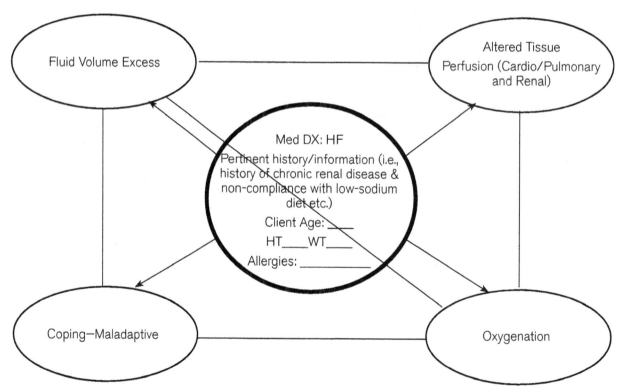

As you can see, all of these concepts are interrelated.

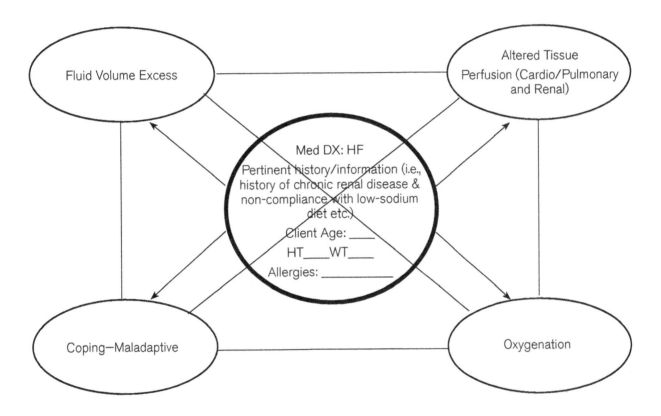

Fluid Volume Excess

Altered Tissue Perfusion (Cardio/Pulmonary and Renal)

Med DX: HF
Pertinent history/information (i.e., history of chronic renal disease & non-compliance with low-sodium diet etc.)
Client Age: ____
HT____WT____
Allergies: _____

Coping—Maladaptive

Oxygenation

> 🖊 *Learning point*: It is important to determine the priority client problems and needs when you are planning care. As a student, you may often want to include anxiety and/or risk for infection on every client's concept map because you may have learned that these concepts are important for the psychosocial and physiological needs. Yes, while it is important for you to assess for anxiety and take steps to prevent infection, only include these on the concept map if the clinical assessment findings support it or if it is a potential complication for the specific client (i.e., client is immunocompromised because they are taking corticosteroids, have a decreased white count, and/or present with a change in the color of the secretions, etc.).

STEP 4: Add System-Specific Assessment Findings

After you have completed your assessment of the client, add the system-specific assessment findings to the concept map. For example:

System-Specific Assessments for Fluid Volume Excess:

Weight 124 lbs. – 4 lb. gain/24 hours

SOB with activity

Lungs clear bilaterally

2+ pitting edema bilaterally in lower legs

Each client's concept you choose will have system-specific assessments that help confirm the hypothesized concepts are correct. It is important to compare the actual system-specific assessment findings with the system-specific assessments that define the concept (Manning & Zager, 2014). As a new graduate nurse, you must be able to not only assess the current clinical findings but be able to anticipate clinical findings that could indicate a potential complication that may occur in the future. These potential complications may be associated with the pathophysiological changes that could occur related to the client's medical diagnoses.

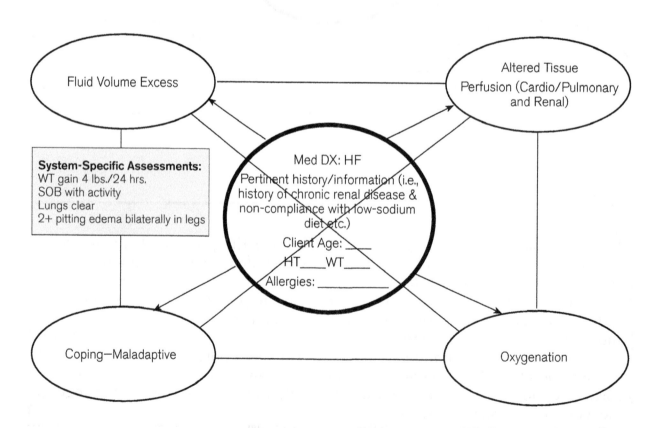

In the assessment findings for oxygenation, the lungs are clear bilaterally. This does not mean that you would stop assessing for adventitious lungs sounds for the client with heart failure who has fluid volume excess. The monitoring, comparing, contrasting, and trending of the clinical assessment findings lead to early identification and/or prevention of potential complications. This competency helps you provide safe and effective care of your client.

Learning Point: After reviewing the system-specific assessment findings, you need to evaluate if you have identified the priority clinical assessment findings for the concept of Fluid Volume Excess. For example, did you include daily weight as a priority clinical assessment finding? We hope you remembered that monitoring the daily weight is the best method of determining fluid status in a client (Manning & Zager, 2014).

Assuming you have included the priority clinical assessment findings, ask yourself the following inquiry questions:

1. *"What clinical findings indicate that my client may have fluid volume excess?"*

2. If you noted that your client gained 4 lbs. ask yourself, *"Was this a weight gain over the past week or in the past 24 hours?"*

Let's assume, for learning purposes, that you do not know. Your next question would be:

3. *"Why is it important for me to know if my client gained or lost weight in the past 24 hours?"*

Using these inquiry questions and seeking the answers, you learn that a 4-lb. weight gain in 24 hours is a significant clinical finding for the concept of fluid volume excess. Repeat this process for all of the concepts you identified on the concept map.

STEP 5: Determine Expected Outcomes and Outcome/Evaluation Criteria

Determining expected outcomes and outcome/evaluation criteria can be very difficult for you because you do not have a lot of clinical experience yet. Do not be discouraged if you struggle with outcome-focused thinking. High level clinical reasoning takes practice (Pesut & Herman, 1999). Here is an easy way to develop outcomes. Transform the concept into a positive term. For example, let's take the concept of fluid volume excess. Ask yourself, "What is the expected outcome for a client with fluid volume excess?" The answer is the client will have fluid volume balance ... voila the **OUTCOME**!

The next step is to determine if the expected outcome was met and if so, how do you know it was met? You develop evaluation criteria using the same process you used for the system-specific assessments and transform them into expected outcomes. For example, one of the assessments for excess fluid volume is *weight gain of 4 pounds since yesterday*. The expected outcome can be measured by the evaluation criteria of *weight gain < 2 lbs. per day*.

The following table illustrates the outcome and evaluation criteria development process for all of the concepts used in this example.

DETERMINE OUTCOMES AND OUTCOME/EVALUATION CRITERIA TABLE

Concepts	System-Specific Assessments	Outcome	Outcome/Evaluation Criteria
Fluid Volume Excess	• Weight gain of 4 lbs. from yesterday • Lungs clear • SOB with activity • 2+ pitting edema bilaterally lower peripheral extremities	Fluid Volume Balance	• Weight gain < 2 lbs./day • Lungs clear • No SOB • No edema bilaterally
Oxygenation	• c/o of SOB • c/o of anxiety • Respirations 23/minute • O_2 Sat 91%	Adequate Oxygenation	• No SOB • No c/o of anxiety • Respirations 16–20/min • O_2 Sat > 95%
Perfusion–Cardiac/Peripheral/Renal	• Capillary refill > 3 sec • Pulses + 1 • Heart rate 88 bpm • Urine 50mL/hr	Adequate Tissue Perfusion	• Capillary refill < 3 sec • Pulses +2 • HR 60–100 bpm • Urine > 30mL/hr
Coping–Maladaptive	• Spouse recently died • Buying processed prepared food for meals • High intake of salt due to processed prepared food • No interest in preparing own meals	Coping–Adaptive	• Met with nutritionist • Connected with grief support group • Able to identify foods with high Na^+ content • Demonstrates interest in preparing own meals

(Manning & Zager, 2014)

STEP 6: Determine Priority Interventions

Determining the priority interventions for the client is the next step. The nursing interventions *italicized* in the the chart of Developing Outcomes And Outcome/Evaluation Criteria With Interventions on page 56 are priority because they help achieve more than one client outcome. The other interventions are distinct to that particular concept and outcome.

When you see all of the interventions on a concept map, you will be able to determine which interventions will be most effective for the most outcomes. This exercise helps you see the client as a whole (system thinking) versus looking at each client's concept and outcome separately (linear thinking). Using the same client, the table illustrates this process with the four concepts used.

Learning Point: Ask yourself these questions to help understand why a particular intervention will help achieve the outcome. For example, the assessment finding of 3+ pitting edema bilaterally in the lower peripheral extremities indicates the need for further interventions.

1. *"What intervention will help decrease peripheral edema?"* You should think about the intervention of positioning.

2. *"What position will best help the client decrease edema?"* We hope this question would prompt you to think about elevating the legs to the level of the heart to help decrease peripheral edema.

3. Another question could be: *"Which of the medications that my client is taking will assist in achieving the expected outcome of fluid balance?"* I bet you immediately thought of diuretics!

DEVELOPING OUTCOMES AND EVALUATION CRITERIA WITH INTERVENTIONS

The italicized interventions are priority because they help achieve more than one client outcome.

Concepts	System-Specific Assessments	Outcome	Outcome/ Evaluation Criteria	Priority Interventions
Fluid Volume Excess	• Weight gain of 4 lbs. from yesterday • Lungs clear • SOB with activity • 2+ pitting edema bilaterally lower peripheral extremities	Fluid Volume Balance	• Weight gain < 2 lbs./day • Lungs clear • No SOB • No edema bilaterally	• Weigh daily, compare & trend • Assess I & O q 8 hrs. • *Assess lung sounds* • *Cough and deep breathe q 4 hrs.* • *Incentive spirometer every hour while awake* • *Semi-Fowler's position with legs elevated at heart level* • *Assess SOB q 4 hrs.* • *Assess edema q 4 hrs.*
Oxygen-ation	• c/o of SOB • c/o of anxiety • Respirations 23/ minute • O_2 Sat 91% with 2L O_2/Nasal cannula • Lungs clear bilaterally	Adequate Oxygenation	• No SOB • Lungs clear • Respirations 16–20/min • O_2 Sat > 95%	• Assess SOB • Assess for restlessness • Assess RR and O_2 sat • Administer O_2 as ordered • *Assess lung sounds* • *Cough and deep breathe q 4 hrs.* • *Incentive spirometer every hour while awake* • *Semi-Fowler's position*
Perfusion— Cardiac/ Peripheral/ Renal	• Capillary refill > 3 sec • Pulses +1 • Heart rate 88 bpm • Urine 50 mL/hr	Adequate Perfusion –Cardiac/ Peripheral/ Renal	• Capillary refill < 3 sec • Pulses +2 bilaterally • Skin warm and dry • Color pink • HR 60–100 bpm • Urine > 30 mL/hr	• Assess capillary refill q 4 hrs. • Assess HR, pulses bilaterally, color & skin temp q 4 hrs. • *Position with legs at heart level* • *HOB Semi-Fowler's position* • Report urine output < 30 mL/ hr or trending ↓
Coping— Maladaptive	• Spouse recently died • Buying processed prepared food for meals • No interest in preparing own meals • High intake of salt due to processed prepared food	Coping– Adaptive	• Collaborative–met with nutritionist • Connected with grief support group • Demonstrates an interest in preparing own meals • Able to identify sources of high Na^+ foods	• Consult to dietary • Assist client in selecting low sodium food from the menu • Consult to grief support group or spiritual advisor

(Manning & Zager, 2014)

STEP 7: Evaluate Outcomes and Make Clinical Judgments About the Plan of Care

The next step is to determine if outcomes have been achieved. This is not a yes or no answer, but a process of comparing, contrasting, and trending the outcome/evaluation criteria to the client's current system-specific assessments. There are three clinical judgments that are possible.

+ Outcome met

+ Outcome partially met

+ Outcome not met

Now that a decision about outcome achievement has been made, you need to decide what the plan of care will be. What are your nursing responsibilities? This is clinical judgment. Clinical judgment requires a series of reflective questions and decisions to plan future client care as indicated in the questions below.

OUTCOME NOT MET

1. Did the client's situation change (i.e., developed adventitious lung sounds)?
    a. If yes, revise plan of care to correspond to the new client condition.
    b. If no, go on to the next question.
2. Did the interventions fail to be effective?
    a. If yes, revise the interventions.
    b. If no, go on to the next question.
3. Did I evaluate too soon or is more time needed for the interventions to be effective?
    a. If yes, continue the current care and continue to evaluate.
    b. If no, go to next question.
4. Were the conclusions drawn from the system-specific assessment findings accurate?
    a. If yes, continue the current plan of care and continue to evaluate.
    b. If no, re-analyze the system-specific assessment findings to determine correct client concept and outcome, and revise the plan of care.

OUTCOME PARTIALLY ACHIEVED

If the outcome was partially achieved, then you would use similar reflection questions.

1. Is more time needed for the interventions to be effective?
   a. If yes, continue the current plan of care and continue to evaluate.
   b. If no, go to next question.
2. Are changes needed in the interventions to achieve the outcome?
   a. If yes, make the changes (i.e., increase the frequency of the interventions or add new interventions, etc.).
   b. If no, continue plan of care and ongoing evaluation.

OUTCOME ACHIEVED

1. Is the problem likely to recur without nursing interventions?
   a. If no, discontinue plan of care.
   b. If yes, go to next question.
2. Does the concept require the same level of intervention or vigilance?
   a. If yes, continue plan of care.
   b. If no, revise plan of care to meet current client needs.

You might be thinking that "The client does not have this concept as a problem because they have no system-specific assessments to confirm the concept, so I need to take it off the concept map."

Reflect for a moment about what you know about heart failure. Based on the pathophysiology of the disease process there is high risk of recurrence of fluid volume excess in a client with heart failure (HF) and renal failure. *It would not be safe practice to quit monitoring for the clinical findings of fluid volume excess even if the client's weight is stable and the lungs are clear. The problem is likely to recur due to the pathophysiological changes that occur with heart failure.* You as a prudent nurse will continue to monitor for potential complications. Therefore, fluid volume excess would remain on the concept map. Here are two examples of inquiry questions to help guide you in this judgment process:

1. *"Your client has HF with renal failure; what is the risk that fluid volume excess may recur?"*
2. *"What would you want to continue to monitor to prevent complications?"*

STEP 8: Document Care Given and Client Response

After making your clinical judgment about your care, you will need to document your conclusions in the medical record. The concept map is a useful guide for you while you document. It is important that the documentation contain the following information:

+ Client's system-specific assessments.

+ Client's response to priority interventions.

+ Progress toward the expected outcomes.

+ Any changes in the plan of care.

The concept map and your clinical notes should provide all of the information you need to document accurately.

PUT THE CONCEPT MAP INTO CLINICAL PRACTICE

The table below, **Putting the Concept Map into Clinical Practice**, describes how you can apply the concept map in the care of your client.

PUTTING THE CONCEPT MAP INTO CLINICAL PRACTICE

Student Responsibility	Learning Points
1. Hypothesize the concepts around the assigned client's medical diagnosis(es) and bring your concept map to clinical.	• Does the concept map reflect the prototype client for this medical diagnosis(es)? If so, go to number 3 under Student Responsibility. • *Remember that the concept map will not have individualized care at this point.*
2. If your hypothesized concepts are incorrect after speaking with your clinical instructor, then edit or add to the concept map. *Hint: Initially use a pencil to complete concept map. Use different color pencil/ ink for different concepts. DO NOT ERASE; just put an X through the revision or change colors, so you can see the CHANGE in THINKING and LEARN from this. Do not start over! This reflects your ability to clinically reason.*	• It is important to remind yourself that what you did the night before or before your clinical day started was not a waste of time. The work provides a basis for your initial system-specific assessments of their client. • Determine if the selected concepts are correct or if there are additional concepts that are a priority to meet the needs of the client.
3. Assess your client and revise concept map as appropriate.	• If after the initial assessment of the client, you need to make revisions in the concept map, remember this is part of the process.

For your reference, at the end of this chapter is an **Example of Adult Health Concept Map** (Appendix A), a **Rubric Grading Tool for the Adult Health Concept Map Example** (Appendix B), and a blank **Adult Health Concept Map Tool** (Appendix C). The rubric will be adjusted based on the level of the course you are taking. For example, in children and family, it would be important to include developmental levels expected for the client's age according to Piaget and Erickson and to evaluate if you understand how to correctly calculate hourly fluid requirements. Maternal and newborn would need to include evaluation of assessment of the mother, fetus, and newborn during and post-delivery.

Additional clinical forms that we have found helpful and can be adapted to your needs are: **AIDES Medication Information Tool** (Appendix D), **Reflection Questions Example** (Appendix E), **History and Pathophysiology Information Tool** (Appendix F), **Health History and System-Specific Assessment Tool** (Appendix G), and **Lab and Diagnostic Tests and Procedures Tool** (Appendix H).

EXAMPLE OF ADULT HEALTH CONCEPT MAP

Name _____ Clinical Faculty _____ Sec # _____ Date _____ Grade _____

Medical DX:
Heart Failure
History of chronic renal & non-compliance with low-sodium diet
Client Age: 68 HT: 5'8"
WT: 184 lbs.
Allergies: NKA

Concept: Perfusion Cardiac/Peripheral/Renal
Outcome: Adequate Perfusion Cardiac/Peripheral/Renal

System-Specific Assessments	Priority Interventions	Outcome/Evaluation Criteria
Cap refill > 3 sec	Assess capillary refill q 4 hrs.	Capillary refill < 3 sec
Pulses + 1 bilaterally	Assess HR, pulses bilaterally, color & skin temp q 4 hrs.	Pulses + 2 bilaterally, HR 60 – 100 bpm; HR & RR return to client's baseline within 3 min after activity
HR–88 bpm	HOB at Semi-Fowler's position with legs at heart level	Skin warm and dry, color pink
Urine 50 mL/hr	Report urine < 30mL/ hr trending ↓	Urine output > 30 mL/hr

Meds R/T to Concept: Digoxin
Labs R/T to Concept: Digoxin level, BUN/Creat
Equipment R/T to Concept: N/A
Client/Family Teaching R/T to Concept: Teach client how to position with lying, sitting or standing to avoid constriction of blood flow & how to monitor HR & RR before & after activity.

Concept: Oxygenation
Outcome: Adequate Oxygenation

System-Specific Assessments	Priority Interventions	Outcome/Evaluation Criteria
c/o of SOB	HOB ↑ semi-Fowler's	No c/o of SOB
R–23/min	C & DB q 4 hrs	RR–16 to 20/min
Lungs clear bilaterally	Incentive spirometer q 1 hr while awake	Lungs clear bilaterally
O_2 Sat 91%	Assess lungs sounds, RR & O_2 Sat q 4 hrs. & PRN & before & after activity	O_2 Sat > 95%
c/o of anxiety	O_2 /Nasal cannula /order	

Meds R/T to Concept:
Labs R/T to Concept: ABGs
Equipment R/T to Concept: O_2 sat monitor, O_2, nasal cannula, incentive spirometer
Client/ Family Teaching R/T to Concept: Instruct how positioning with HOB↑ expands lung capacity.

Concept: Coping—Maladaptive
Outcome: Coping—Adaptive

System-Specific Assessments	Priority Interventions	Outcome/Evaluation Criteria
Spouse recently died	Consult to dietary	Met with dietician
Buying processed prepared food for meals	Assist client in selecting low-sodium food from the menu	Connected with grief support group or spiritual adviser
High intake of Na+ due to processed foods	Consult to grief support group	Able to identify foods with low Na+ content from list
No interest in preparing own meals		Able to plan menu with low-Na+ foods

Meds R/T to Concept:
Labs R/T to Concept:
Equipment R/T to Concept:
Client/Family Teaching R/T to Concept: Dietary consult related to selecting low-Na+ foods, grief support and group or spiritual advisor to assist with coping

Date_____

Concept: Fluid Volume Excess
Outcome: Fluid Volume Balance

System-Specific Assessments	Priority Interventions	Outcome/Evaluation Criteria
Wt. 124 lbs – 4-lbs. gain/24 hrs	I & O q 8 hrs. Weigh daily, compare & trend	Wt gain < 2lbs/day
SOB with activity	↑ legs when sitting/lying (at level of heart)	No c/o of SOB
Lungs clear bilaterally	Incentive spirometer q 1 hr while awake	Lungs clear bilaterally
2+ pitting edema bilaterally in lower legs	Assess lungs sounds, RR, SOB & O_2 Sat q 4 hrs. & PRN, trend	No edema bilaterally

Meds R/T to Concept: Furosemide
Labs R/T to Concept: Electrolytes, particularly K+, Na+ level, BUN/Creat
Equipment R/T to Concept: Scales
Client/Family Teaching R/T to Concept: Dietary consult related to selecting low-sodium foods

To be completed and reviewed the day of clinical by: Clinical Instructor signature: _____

cont'd on next page

EXAMPLE OF ADULT HEALTH CONCEPT MAP   PAGE 2

Name_____

Evaluation of Outcome Criteria: Perfusion	Rationale for Interventions:	Client response to interventions:
• HR ↑ 98 bpm with activity, returns to resting pulse < 3 min • Cap refill remains > 3min • Pulses remain 1+ bilaterally • Urine output 320 mL/8 hrs. = > 40 mL/hr	Urine output > 30 mL/hr indicates adequate perfusion to the kidneys. Increase in HR & RR that does not return to client's normal within 3 min indicates an increase workload on the heart with resulting decrease in oxygen provided to vital organs.	Client positioned in bed with HOB elevated and legs elevated at heart level when lying. Having difficulty prioritizing activity so HR & RR return to baseline within 3 min.

Clinical Judgment. Was overall outcome met? Yes ____ Partially __x__ Not at all ____
Rationale: Explain your decision. What would you do differently? Progress is being made but because of disease processes of HF, will continually need to monitor and pace activities with rest periods as client tolerates. Teach client to pace activities. Continue plan of care.

Evaluation of Outcome Criteria: Oxygenation	Rationale for Interventions:	Client response to interventions:
• Client states SOB is better with activity • RR decreased from 23 to 20/min • Lungs remain clear bilaterally • O₂ sat 94% on 2L O₂ via NC	Elevation of HOB allows chest expansion, promotes oxygenation. Incentive spirometer helps client take long deep breaths, O₂/NC has increased O₂ sat, need to continue to monitor O₂ sat.	Client stated ↓SOB and was able to breathe easier with the O₂ and the HOB elevated.

Clinical Judgment. Was overall outcome met? Yes ____ Partially __x__ Not at all ____
Rationale: Explain your decision. What would you do differently? Client made significant improvement as indicated by decrease RR and increased O₂ sat, but needs to continue plan of care until able to keep O₂ Sat > 95% on 2 L O₂/NC.

Evaluation of Outcome Criteria: Fluid Balance	Rationale for Interventions:	Client response to interventions:
• No weight gain in 24 hrs. * Decreased SOB with activity * Edema remains at 2+ bilaterally * Lungs remain clear bilaterally	Monitor fluid balance with daily weights and I & O q 8 hrs. because excess fluid volume increases the workload on the heart.	Client verbalizing understanding of how increased Na⁺ content in the diet contributes to excess fluid that makes it difficult to breathe and the heart has to work harder to pump the extra fluid. Keeping legs elevated at heart level when in bed.

Clinical Judgment. Was overall outcome met? Yes ____ Partially __x__ Not at all ____
Rationale: Explain your decision. What would you do differently? Client making progress but will need to continue the plan of care. Will recommend a dietary consult to help with teaching about low Na⁺ diets and a physical therapy consult to help teach client exercises to help promote venous circulation and decrease edema in lower legs.

Priority Lab/Procedures	Results/Interpretations	Nursing Indications (Pre & Post)
• Electrolytes, Na⁺ & K⁺ • BUN/Creat	• Na⁺–138 mEq/L K⁺–3.2 mEq/L • BUN 19/Creat 1.9	• Notify healthcare provider prior to giving furosemide because K⁺ is 3.2 mEq/L. • Continue to monitor because of HF and receiving an ace inhibitor.

© 2017 ICAN Publishing Inc. Developed by Lydia R. Zager, MSN, RN, NEA–BC; Additions from Kate Chappell, MSN, APRN, CPNP

RUBRIC GRADING TOOL FOR ADULT HEALTH CONCEPT MAP EXAMPLE

Student Name _____ Faculty _____ Date _____

Directions: Complete one **Concept Map** each week. You will get a Pass/Fail. One of the written concept maps will be graded and one will be presented orally to your clinical instructor on designated weeks. The average of the two will be 5% of your application grade. You will receive your assigned client and primary medical diagnosis(es) when you arrive for clinical, listen to report, do your assessment and then do the first page of the concept map. The concept map is a working tool, so **make appropriate changes/additions throughout the day as the clinical situation dictates. Use a different color ink or pencil to make your changes in the concept map.** Complete the first page of your concept map by the end of clinical for your clinical instructor to review and sign. The final review will be completed when all components of the concept map, AIDES sheets and reflection page are turned in/emailed to your faculty. SBAR will be given as directed or per unit protolcol.

CONCEPT MAP COMPONENTS WITH CRITERIA FOR GRADING	POINTS
1. Identify **3 overall outcomes and their relevant Concept label** based on medical diagnosis & clinical condition. *3 pts for each of 3 appropriate priority concepts x 3 = 9)*	___/9 ___P/F
2. Indicate client findings for **focused (system-specific) assessments for each of the 3 concepts. All key assessments included—minimum of 3 each.** *3 pts for each concept's assessment findings (3 x 3 = 9)*	___/9 ___P/F
3. Identify **specific measurable outcomes for concepts. All outcome criteria incl. to fully address each overall outcome—minimum of 2 each.** *4 pts for the specific outcome criteria per overall outcome (3 x 4 = 12)*	___/12 ___P/F
4. Identify at least **4 priority interventions that will help achieve outcomes: Include at least 2 action interventions** (i.e., cough & deep breathe q 2 hrs.) **& 2 priority assessments** for client's condition/response (i.e, monitor VS q 4 hrs. & compare to previous findings). *(3 x 4 = 12)*	___/4 ___P/F
5. Use **lines to show relationships** between concepts (i.e., there is a pathophysiological connection between the two concepts). Use different colored pencils/pens for each concept to draw the lines to make the relationships clearer. *Points based on relationships being valid.*	___/4 ___P/F
6. On page 1, **indicate appropriate medications and diagnostic results pertinent to each concept.**	___/4 ___P/F
7. On page 1, **indicate appropriate safety/equipment risks/precautions** (fall, seizures, infection control, etc.) and **family involvement/teaching needs for each concept.**	___/4 ___P/F
TOTAL POINTS POSSIBLE	100

CONCEPT MAP COMPONENTS WITH CRITERIA FOR GRADING	POINTS
8. On page 2, **evaluate the client's response** to each intervention & progress toward desired outcomes. *3 pts for accurate evaluation of outcome criteria and interventions for each overall outcome x 3 = 9*	___/9 ___P/F
9. **State if overall outcomes were met. Provide & explain a clinical decision about each outcome based on your evaluation** (i.e., continue, modify, D/C). *3 pts for each overall outcome clinical decision (3 x 3 = 9)*	___/9 ___P/F
10. On page 2, **interpret priority lab/diagnostic values** related to the client's current clinical condition with **nursing indications/care.**	___/6 ___P/F
11. On 3 AIDES medication sheets, **describe 3 medications & identify nursing** indications & desired outcome for the medications. *3 points for each medication*	___/9 ___P/F
12. Complete the History and Pathophysiology Information on the form as directed. Turn in with the concept map.	___/3 ___P/F
13. **Critical Thinking/Reflection Questions** are answered completely & clearly with appropriate detail. Answers reflect a complete understanding of the client situation.	___/6 ___P/F
14. Correctly prepare and give the SBAR report to clinical instructor prior to reporting of to the assigned RN.	___/4 ___P/F
TOTAL POINTS RECEIVED	

APPENDIX C

Chapter 4

ADULT HEALTH CONCEPT MAP TOOL

Name _____ Clinical Instructor _____ Sec # _____ Date _____ Grade _____

Top-left concept box

Concept:
Outcome:

System-Specific Assessments	Priority Interventions	Outcome/Evaluation Criteria

Meds R/T to Concept:
Labs R/T to Concept:
Equipment R/T to Concept:
Client/ Family Teaching R/T to Concept:

Top-right concept box

Concept:
Outcome:

System-Specific Assessments	Priority Interventions	Outcome/Evaluation Criteria

Meds R/T to Concept:
Labs R/T to Concept:
Equipment R/T to Concept:
Client/ Family Teaching R/T to Concept:

Center

Medical DX:
  History:
  Client Age:
  HT: WT:
  Allergies:

Bottom-left concept box

Concept:
Outcome:

System-Specific Assessments	Priority Interventions	Outcome/Evaluation Criteria

Meds R/T to Concept:
Labs R/T to Concept:
Equipment R/T to Concept:
Client/Family Teaching R/T to Concept:

Bottom-right concept box

Concept:
Outcome:

System-Specific Assessments	Priority Interventions	Outcome/Evaluation Criteria

Meds R/T to Concept:
Labs R/T to Concept:
Equipment R/T to Concept:
Client/Family Teaching R/T to Concept:

To be completed and reviewed the day of clinical by: Clinical Instructor signature: _____ Date _____

Developed by Lydia R. Zager, MSN, RN, NEA-BC; Additions from Kate Chappell, MSN, APRN, CPNP

ADULT HEALTH CONCEPT MAP TOOL, PAGE 2

Name _____

Client response to interventions:

Rationale for Interventions:

Evaluation of Outcome Criteria:

Clinical Judgment. Was overall outcome met?   Yes _____   Partially _____   Not at all _____
Rationale: Explain your decision. What would you do differently?

Client response to interventions:

Rationale for Interventions:

Evaluation of Outcome Criteria:

Clinical Judgment. Was overall outcome met?   Yes _____   Partially _____   Not at all _____
Rationale: Explain your decision. What would you do differently?

Client response to interventions:

Rationale for Interventions:

Evaluation of Outcome Criteria:

Clinical Judgment. Was overall outcome met?   Yes _____   Partially _____   Not at all _____
Rationale: Explain your decision. What would you do differently?

Priority Lab/Procedures	Results/Interpretations	Nursing Indications (Pre & Post)

AIDES MEDICATION INFORMATION TOOL

Directions: Please complete on _____ of your priority medications
Turn into clinical instructor _____
Have ready as information for all drugs you are administering (book, drug cards)

"AIDES" to Assist in Remembering Facts for Medication Administration

Name of Drug: Brand_____ **Generic**_____

Classification_____ **Referenced Used**_____

A Action of medication:

Administration of medication. Dosage ordered_____

How to administer:

Assessment:

Adverse Effects. List significant ones:

Accuracy/Appropriateness of order. Is it indicated based on client's condition, known allergies, drug-drug or drug-food interactions? If not, what action did you take?

I Interactions (Drug-Drug, Food-Drug):

Identify priority plan prior to giving drug (i.e., vital signs, labs, allergies, etc.):

Identify priority plan after giving drug:

D Desired outcomes of the drug:

Discharge teaching—Administration considerations for client and family:

E Evaluate signs and symptoms of complications. Intervene if necessary and describe:

S Safety (client identification, risk for falls, vital sign assessments):

EXAMPLE OF REFLECTION QUESTIONS

Student Name _____ Clinical Instructor _____

Sec # _____ Date_____ Sat/UnSat or Grade_____

Date due to Clinical Instructor: _____

Six (6) points are possible and will be added to Rubric Grading Tool for the Concept Map (see Appendix B)

1. Connect the system-specific findings (diagnostic test results) to the priority interventions (medications, treatments) for your client and provide the rationale. (2 points)

2. Based on your analysis of the concepts, what are the expected outcomes for your client? (2 points)

3. What went well today for you in clinical and why? (1 point)

4. What would you do differently and why? (1 point)

HISTORY AND PATHOPHYSIOLOGY INFORMATION TOOL

Student Name _____ Faculty _____ Sec #_____

Date _____   Pass/Fail or Grade_____

Directions: Complete and submit to clinical instructor by _____.
(10 points possible on the Rubric Grading Tool for the Concept Map)

Client's Story (History)—What symptoms required the client to come to the hospital?

PATHOPHYSIOLOGY

Please describe the etiology (cause) and pathophysiology in your words. This is to be completed for the major diagnosis and any other active diagnoses that affect care (i.e., diabetes).

List the signs and symptoms of the disease from the textbook. Compare it to the system-specific assessment findings from your client (may complete the comparison after you care for your client during clinical).

Assessment findings (signs & symptoms)   Assessment findings my client manifested:
from textbook:

_____   _____

_____   _____

_____   _____

_____   _____

_____   _____

_____   _____

_____   _____

HEALTH HISTORY AND SYSTEM-SPECIFIC ASSESSMENT TOOL	
Demographic Information	
Source of History	
Chief Concern/Complaint	
History of Present Illness (HPI)	
Past Medical History (PMH)	
Family History (FH)	
Social History (SH)	
Health Promotion Behaviors	
Review of Systems (ROS) System-Specific as indicated by client condition: • Integument • Head and Neck • Eyes • Ears, Nose, Mouth and Throat • Breasts • Respiratory • Cardiovascular • Gastrointestinal • Genitourinary • Musculoskeletal • Neurological • Mental Health • Endocrine • Allergic/Immunologic	
Focused History of Symptom(s) • Location • Quality • Quantity • Timing • Setting • Alleviating or Aggravating Factors • Associated Phenomenon	

Adapted by Ellen Synovec, MN

cont'd on next page

HEALTH HISTORY AND SYSTEM-SPECIFIC ASSESSMENT TOOL *(cont'd)*

II PHYSICAL ASSESSMENT

General Survey
1. Appearance
2. Level of Consciousness
3. Behavior/Affect
4. Posture/dress
5. Signs of discomfort or distress
6. Assess pupils for symmetry, shape, reactivity light

Skin Assessment:
1. Color
2. Condition—Look behind ears, skin folds, between toes, soles of feet, pressure areas on shoulder, sacrum, heels Presence or absence or lesions, scars, wounds or piercings
3. Texture
4. Temperature
5. Skin turgor sternum
6. Nails condition, presence of clubbing
7. Capillary refill bilaterally fingers

Respiratory Assessment
1. Rate
2. Rhythm
3. Accessory muscle use
4. Chest shape and symmetry/spinal deformities/AP: LA
5. Ausculation 12 sites anterior, posterior and axillary—assess for presence or absence of adventitious sounds, cough, congestion

Cardiac assessment
1. PMI—assess location and size
2. 4 auscultation sites with diaphragm and bell
   a. Aortic—2nd RICS RSB
   b. Pulmonic—2nd LICS LSB
   c. Tricuspid—4th LICS, along left lateral sternal border
   d. Mitral or apical pulse—5th LICS MCL, apex of heart
3. Carotids—assess pulse quality, presence or absence of thrills/bruits, bilaterally
4. JVD
5. Lymph nodes

Abdomen
1. Size
2. Shape
3. Symmetry
4. Condition—presence or absence of piercings, scars, striae, pulsations, peristalsis or bulges
5. Bowel sounds—assess all 4 quads, # sounds per minute RLQ
6. Assess for distention or tenderness with light palpation

Extremities
1. Capillary refill to upper extremities (UE)
2. Assess UE and lower extremities (LE) for general range of motion
3. Assess UE and LE for condition, color, temperature and presence of edema
4. Palpation of peripheral pulses—radial and dorsal pedalis
5. Assess clonus

Adapted by Ellen Synovec, MN

LAB AND DIAGNOSTIC TESTS AND PROCEDURES TOOL
Use as Reference for Client Care

Name: _____

Date: _____

Client Initials: _____

Directions: Identify only <u>pertinent</u> labs to the client condition, whether normal or abnormal. Describe what caused the client to have an abnormal lab or why a lab may now be normal (e.g., norm WBC–client on antibiotics). Also explain why you would or would not call the healthcare provider about this lab. These laboratory values may vary in textbooks. Look at the accepted norms for the institution where the test is interpreted to determine abnormal versus normal. This list is not all inclusive.

Lab Test	Date of Lab Test	Results	Normal	Pertinence to Client	Would You Call the Healthcare Provider?
Hematology					
WBC			5.0 – 10.0 10^3 ul		
RBC			4.2 – 5.4 10^6 µL		
HGB			12.0 – 16.0 g/dL		
HbA1c			6% or less		
HCT			37.0 – 47.0%		
MCV			81 – 89 µm^3		
MCH			26 – 35 pg/cell		
MCHC			31 – 37 g/dl		
Platelets			150,000– 400,000/mm^3		
Neutrophils			37 – 75%		
Lymphocytes			19 – 48%		
Monocytes			0 – 10%		
Eosinophils			1 – 3%		
Basophils			0.0 – 1.5%		
Chemistry					
Sodium			135 – 145 mEq/L		
Potassium			3.5 – 5.1 mEq/L		
Chloride			98 – 107 mEq/L		
Glucose–serum			70 – 110 mg/dL		
Magnesium			1.3 – 2.1 mEq/L		
BUN			6 – 20 mg/dL		
Creatinine			0.7 – 1.4 mg/dL		
Calcium			8.5 –11.0 mg/dL		
Protein			6.0 – 8.0 mg/dL		
Albumin			3.5 – 5.0 mg/dL		
A/G Ratio			1.5:1.0 – 2.5 :1.0		
Total Bilirubin			0.3 –1.3 mg/dL		
Direct bilirubin			0 – 0.4 mg/dL		
Indirect Bilirubin			0.2 – .8 mg/dL		
ALT, SGPT			10 – 30 U/L		
AST, SGOT			8 – 46 U/L		
Ammonia			80 – 110 dL/mcg		

cont'd on next page

APPENDIX H

LAB AND DIAGNOSTIC TESTS AND PROCEDURES TOOL *(cont'd)*

Lab Test	Date of Lab Test	Results	Normal	Pertinence to Client	Would You Call the Healthcare Provider?
LDH – serum			91 – 180 mg/dL		
Alk Phos			35 – 142 U/L		
Uric Acid			2 – 7 mg/dL		
Phosphorus			2.5 – 4.5 mg/dL		
Total Cholesterol			< 200 mg/dL		
LDL age > 45 (LD)			90 – 185 mg/dL		
HDL			40 – 65 mg/dL		
Triglyceride			35 – 150 mg/dL		
Urinalysis					
Color			Clear Yellow		
Appearance			Clear		
Glucose			Neg.		
Bilirubin			Neg		
Ketones			Neg		
Specific Gravity			1.015 – 1.025		
Blood			Neg		
Ph			5 – 9		
Protein			Neg		
Urobilinogen			0.5 – 4.0 mg/24hr		
Nitrates			Neg		
ABG's					
pH			7.35 – 7.45		
pCO_2			35 – 45 mm Hg		
pO_2			80 – 100 mm Hg		
HCO_3			22 – 26 mEq /L		
O_2 Sat			> 95%		
Type of O_2 client receiving					
Digoxin			0.5 – 2.0 µg/mL		
Dilantin			10 – 20 µg/mL		
Tegretol			4 – 12 µg/mL		
Theophylline			10 – 20 µg/mL		
Pt			12 – 14 SEC		
Ptt			30 – 45 SEC		
Amylase			25 – 125 U/dL		
Cardiac Enzymes					
Myoglobin			30 – 90 ng/mL		
Total CPK (CK)			Male 5 – 55 U/L Female 5 – 25 U/L		
CPK-MB			0 – 7% of total CPK		
CPK-BB			0% of total CPK		
CPK-MM			5 – 70% of total CPK		
Troponin I Value			< 0.6 ng/mL		
BNP			< 100 pg/mL		

LAB AND DIAGNOSTIC TESTS AND PROCEDURES TOOL *(cont'd)*

DIAGNOSTIC TESTS/PROCEDURES

1. X-Ray, Endoscopy, Scans, Biopsy, C & S, or other special procedure reports

   Test: _____

   Date: _____

   Conclusion/Interpretations: _____

   _____

   _____

   Pertinence to Client: _____

2. X-Ray, Endoscopy, Scans, Biopsy, C&S, or other special procedure reports

   Test: _____

   Date: _____

   Conclusion/Interpretations: _____

   _____

   _____

   Pertinence to Client: _____

3. X-Ray, Endoscopy, Scans, Biopsy, C & S, or other special procedure reports

   Test: _____

   Date: _____

   Conclusion/Interpretations: _____

   _____

   _____

   Pertinence to Client: _____

ENGAGING THE LEARNER ACTIVITIES

Chapter 4

STUDENT-CENTERED LEARNING ACTIVITIES
LINKED TO PROFESSIONAL AND NCLEX® STANDARDS

Resources Needed for Activities	*Concepts Made Insanely Easy for Clinical Nursing* (Manning & Zager, 2014); *The Eight-Step Approach for Student Clinical Success* (Zager, Manning & Herman, 2018)
Standards	**Student Instructions**
Management of Care Plan, implement, and evaluate client-centered care based on Standards of Practice.	**Steps in Constructing the Concept Map** (Refer to Chapter 4 and *Concepts Made Insanely Easy for Clinical Nursing* for concepts, assessments, and expected outcomes) 1. Construct a concept map. a. Proceed step by step as listed in this chapter. b. Ask questions as needed about the steps as you construct the concept map.
Management of Care Plan, implement, and evaluate client-centered care based on Standards of Practice.	**Concept Map Practice** (Refer to the **Adult Health Concept Map Tool** (Appendix C) and the book *Concepts Made Insanely Easy for Clinical Nursing* for concepts, assessments, and expected outcomes) 2. Based on the assigned disease or pathophysiological process, construct a concept map with your partner. a. Hypothesize possible concepts related to the pathophysiology of the disease process. b. Determine what assessments would confirm or reject your hypothesized concepts. c. Select the priority interventions after you analyze the concepts. d. Determine the outcome criteria that would indicate your client has met the expected outcomes.

Mastering Clinical Concepts

IN THIS CHAPTER YOU WILL:

➤ Analyze priority concepts

➤ Determine priority interventions

➤ Evaluate expected outcomes

➤ Identify related priority concepts

When you get your clinical assignment do you ask yourself, "What do I do now?" Do you feel overwhelmed with the mountains of information in your medical surgical and other textbooks? Graduate nurses are expected to learn and retain volumes of information in order to give prioritized quality care.

In the previous chapter, you learned how to do a concept map. In this chapter, we will show you how to use the "SAFETY" model (Refer to Chapter 3, "SAFETY" Model, Appendix A) to connect the pathophysiology of the disease your client is presenting with to the priority concepts, including the assessments, interventions, and expected outcomes. When you get your client's diagnosis, you need to determine what system or systems are involved. Using the information from your textbooks, you connect the system-specific pathophysiology of the disease to the concepts. Once you learn the concepts, you will know what to do!

ANALYZE PRIORITY CONCEPTS

Concepts are a way of chunking information in phases that help us communicate with each other and the healthcare team. For example, perfusion means the heart is pumping adequately through the arteries and capillaries to all organs and tissues delivering oxygen, nutrients, and removing cellular waste. If there is no perfusion or inadequate perfusion, it results in tissue injury, and ultimately the death of tissues and organs (Manning & Zager, 2014, p. 155). When we say the word perfusion to each other, we know what it means. That is why learning concepts is a very efficient way to prioritize nursing care.

Every time you talk about a concept, you need to know how to measure it. Let's take cardiac perfusion. How do you know the heart is perfusing?

If the heart does not perfuse adequately, your system-specific assessments may include:

+ Capillary refill maybe > 3 seconds.

+ Heart rate may increase or decrease.

+ Respirations may increase.

+ Skin color may be pale.

+ Extremities may be cool.

+ May have decrease in O_2 saturation.

+ Urine output may decrease.

+ May have pain (chest or peripheral).

+ Pulses may be weak or thready.

These system-specific assessments apply to all medical conditions affecting cardiac perfusion, (i.e., hypertension, atherosclerosis, peripheral vascular disease) that are caused by constriction or obstruction. Then there can be medical conditions such as heart failure, cardiomyopathy, valvular heart disease, and cardiac arrhythmias that are a result of mechanical and electrical conduction which cause an alteration in the cardiac output. Rheumatic heart disease, endocarditis, myocarditis, and pericarditis are caused from infections and inflammation (Manning & Zager, 2014, p. 156). Refer to **The Pathophysiology Behind a Decrease in Cardiac/Peripheral Perfusion** (Appendix A).

The mnemonic "PUMPS", outlined in **Linking Pathophysiology to System-Specific Assessments for Cardiac and Peripheral Perfusion** (Appendix B), is an EASY way to remember the system-specific assessments for cardiac perfusion (Manning & Zager, 2014, p. 160). Note the left column in Appendix B is the pathophysiology that results in the system-specific assessments in the right column.

Mastering the concepts allows you to become confident in your ability to know what system-specific assessments and data are necessary to collect. With this mastery, you will be able to recognize trends in the clinical findings that indicate a potential complication.

DETERMINE PRIORITY INTERVENTIONS

The priority nursing concept in the example above is "decreased perfusion." The priority nursing interventions with decreased cardiac perfusion include:

+ Position the head of the bed correctly.

+ Evaluate vital signs and pulses.

+ Report trends indicating a decrease in urine output.

+ Report trends in fluid management.

+ Manage energy conservation.

+ Use support stockings or intermittent compression devices.

+ Encourage ambulation (except if there is chest pain, an infection of the heart, severe heart failure, or cardiomyopathy, then bedrest is required).

The mnemonic "**PERFUSE**", outlined in **Linking Pathophysiology to Interventions for Cardiac/Peripheral Perfusion "PERFUSE"** (Appendix C), is an EASY way to remember the priority interventions for cardiac perfusion (Manning & Zager, 2014, p. 164). Note the left column in Appendix C is the pathophysiology that results in the first-do priority Interventions in the right column.

By using the structure of the "SAFETY" model, we have eliminated large volumes of information often seen in nursing textbooks. The structure of the "SAFETY" model is based on standards (i.e., patient safety, practice, QSEN, and NCLEX®) and focuses on the priority information that is *"necessary to know versus nice to know."* Also, the "SAFETY" model will assist you in developing clinical decision making skills.

EVALUATE EXPECTED OUTCOMES

How do you know if your priority nursing interventions were effective? You assess the client for system-specific assessments that indicate the expected outcome(s) were met within the defined limits of your client. Has the client gotten better, stayed the same or gotten worse? Note in the **SAFETY Summary: Concept Cardiac/Peripheral Perfusion** (Appendix D) that the evaluation is simply reviewing the initial system-specific assessments and determining if the assessments and/or lab values have returned to the client's defined limits (Manning & Zager, 2014, p.165).

IDENTIFY RELATED PRIORITY CONCEPTS

During any assessment of your client, you may assess new clinical findings. If you do, ask yourself, "What do these new assessments mean?" Often the clinical findings may indicate a related concept(s) based on the pathophysiological process. Let's look at an example. Your client who had alteration in cardiac perfusion now has the following system-specific assessment findings:

+ Respiratory rate has increased to 26/min.

+ Lungs have adventitious sounds bilaterally.

+ O_2 saturation has decreased to 92%.

+ Complaint of shortness of breath (SOB).

+ Temperature equal to or greater than 101.9°F.

+ Expectorating small amounts of pale-yellow secretions.

Through your analysis of the system-specific assessment findings, you have identified these are associated with the respiratory system. Your new related priority concept is **alteration in oxygenation**. As you review the results from the system-specific labs and diagnostic procedures (i.e., ABGs, CBC, sputum cultures, and chest x-ray) you note the healthcare provider concluded the client now has pneumonia. You will note the pathophysiology is due to a lower respiratory tract infection as indicated in **The Pathophysiology Behind Alterations in Oxygenation** (Appendix E), (Manning & Zager, 2014, p. 124).

As with the concept of perfusion, we have provided you with an EASY way to remember the concept of Oxygenation:

+ Refer to "DYSPNEA" in **Linking Pathophysiology to System-Specific Assessments for Altered Oxygenation** (Appendix F), (Manning & Zager, 2014, p. 125).

+ Refer to "BREATHE" in **Linking Pathophysiology to First-Do-Priority Interventions for Altered Oxygenation** (Appendix G), (Manning & Zager, 2014, p. 130).

+ Refer to the **SAFETY Summary: Concept Oxygenation** (Appendix H) to review evaluation of expected outcomes for clients with alteration in oxygenation (Manning & Zager, 2014, p. 131).

By using the "SAFETY" Model, you have been able to determine other physiological concepts that are impacting your client and require additional interventions. Mastering concepts allows you to apply the information to other clients with different disease processes. The concepts of perfusion and oxygenation, for example, are the same for a client with respiratory, renal, or neuro, etc. disease processes with only a few minor exceptions. At the same time, you are following the standards necessary for both NCLEX® and clinical success (Refer to Chapter 8).

The book *Medical Surgical Nursing Concepts Made Insanely Easy: A New Approach to Prioritization* presents a revolutionary approach to using concepts and managing volumes of information in a way you can learn and remember. This book is an excellent resource to assist you in mastering numerous concepts and priority nursing care and is written within the framework of NCLEX® standards, "SAFETY" Model and prioritization.

THE PATHOPHYSIOLOGY BEHIND
A DECREASE IN CARDIAC/PERIPHERAL PERFUSION

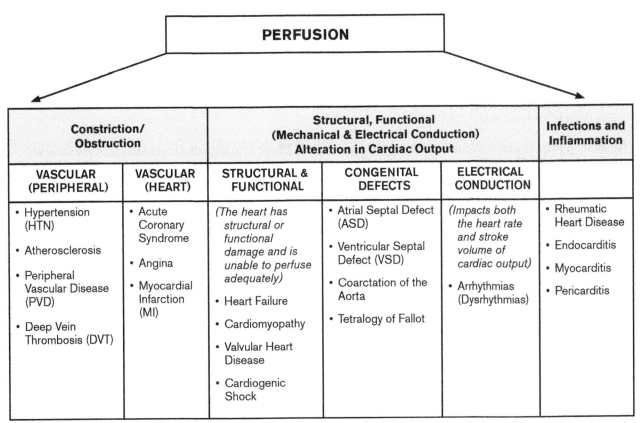

PERFUSION					
Constriction/ Obstruction		**Structural, Functional (Mechanical & Electrical Conduction) Alteration in Cardiac Output**			**Infections and Inflammation**
VASCULAR (PERIPHERAL)	**VASCULAR (HEART)**	**STRUCTURAL & FUNCTIONAL**	**CONGENITAL DEFECTS**	**ELECTRICAL CONDUCTION**	
• Hypertension (HTN) • Atherosclerosis • Peripheral Vascular Disease (PVD) • Deep Vein Thrombosis (DVT)	• Acute Coronary Syndrome • Angina • Myocardial Infarction (MI)	*(The heart has structural or functional damage and is unable to perfuse adequately)* • Heart Failure • Cardiomyopathy • Valvular Heart Disease • Cardiogenic Shock	• Atrial Septal Defect (ASD) • Ventricular Septal Defect (VSD) • Coarctation of the Aorta • Tetralogy of Fallot	*(Impacts both the heart rate and stroke volume of cardiac output)* • Arrhythmias (Dysrhythmias)	• Rheumatic Heart Disease • Endocarditis • Myocarditis • Pericarditis

(Manning, L. & Zager, L. (2014). Medical surgical nursing concepts made insanely easy! A new approach to prioritization, Duluth, GA: ICAN Publishing, Inc., p. 156.)

APPENDIX B

LINKING PATHOPHYSIOLOGY TO SYSTEM-SPECIFIC ASSESSMENTS FOR CARDIAC/PERIPHERAL PERFUSION

Pathophysiology	System-Specific Assessments
Pulses: The heart sounds, S_1 and S_2 indicate that the heart is pumping and the cardiac conduction system is working. S_3 and S_4 are abnormal heart sounds but may be present if the client has heart failure or hypertension *(refer to heart sounds on previous page for specifics).* Palpable peripheral pulses indicate the body and the extremities are receiving adequate perfusion. A client that is alert and responsive indicates there is perfusion to the brain.	**P**ulses (peripheral and JVD) assess bilaterally and compare, capillary refill $>$ 3 seconds, auscultate heart sounds (presence of S_3 or S_4), heart rate, rhythm, (pulse $\downarrow$ or $\uparrow$ with arrhythmias), and BP. Assess for $\downarrow$ level of consciousness (LOC), syncope.
Urine output $>$ 30 mL/hour is an indication that the kidneys are being perfused. The kidneys are affected early with decreased perfusion. If there is a decrease urine output and the body is retaining fluid, the excess fluid requires the heart to pump harder *(Refer to concept Fluid & Electrolytes for specifics).*	**U**rine output ($<$ 30 mL/hour), I & O, and daily weights. Compare, contrast, and trend all.
Moist lung sounds (adventitious) and edema. A client with heart failure or PVD may have edema or adventitious lung sounds present because the pumping action of the heart is not adequate to either return blood to the heart or pump blood to the body. This in combination with excess fluid leads to decreased oxygenation.	**M**oist lung sounds (adventitious), $\uparrow$ RR, check O_2 sat; edema (compare R & L extremities).
Pain: Chest pain is caused by inadequate oxygen to the heart muscle. Decreased perfusion = decreased oxygenation = chest pain *(Refer to angina and chest pain in this chapter).* Chest pain could indicate there is an increased workload demand on the heart. This could result from activity, medications, and/or increased heart rate. That in turn causes ischemia (chest pain) from inadequate perfusion. If there is decreased perfusion to the extremities with peripheral artery disease (PAD), the client experiences intermittent claudication, which is also pain from ischemia *(Refer to PAD in this chapter for specifics).*	**P**ain will vary *(refer to angina, MI, PVD for specifics).* Assess to see if pain increases with activity.
Skin Color: Pale skin and cool temperature may indicate a decrease in perfusion. Temperature elevations may occur with infections of the heart *(Refer to Infections in this chapter)* or valve disease *(Refer to Valve disorders in this chapter for specifics).*	**S**kin Color: pale, cool extremities, $\uparrow$ temp (for infections of the heart or heart valves disorders

(Manning, L. & Zager, L. (2014). Medical surgical nursing concepts made insanely easy! A new approach to prioritization, Duluth, GA: ICAN Publishing, Inc., p. 160.)

LINKING PATHOPHYSIOLOGY TO INTERVENTIONS
FOR CARDIAC/PERIPHERAL PERFUSION "PERFUSE"

Pathophysiology	First-Do Priority Interventions
Position: A decrease in perfusion = decrease in oxygenation to the organs and tissues. Positioning client in an upright position helps facilitate the expansion of the lungs for adequate oxygenation *(Refer to concept Oxygenation for specifics)*. If the client's BP has decreased, semi-Fowler's to supine position will increase perfusion. Remember with decreased perfusion, you want to position the client to avoid constriction of blood flow and promote oxygenation. Cold and nicotine both cause vasoconstriction.	**P**osition HOB ↑. NOTE: if BP decreases, lower HOB to semi-Fowler's or supine position *(Refer to PVD for specifics on positioning)*. Give supplement O2 as needed. Avoid restrictive clothes, cold, and nicotine.
Evaluate: Assessments can change quickly (i.e., pulmonary edema, myocardial infarction, and arrhythmias). Comparing, contrasting, and trending assessments will indicate if there is decreased cardiac and peripheral perfusion or if the client is not adequately oxygenating. The evaluation of the healing of an incision site with clients who have had surgical procedures (i.e., coronary bypass surgery, valve replacements, pacemaker insertions, etc.) will indicate if there is adequate perfusion to the wound. Decreased perfusion to the incision site can delay wound healing.	**E**valuate VS, pulses, edema (compare R & L extremities), lung sounds, ECG, CVP, and hemodynamic monitoring. Evaluate surgical incision site: bleeding, skin temp, circulation, color, signs of infection, and healing.
Report Urine Output: The hourly urine output is an indication of the perfusion of the kidneys. A heart with failure or damage to the muscle or valves is unable to adequately perfuse vital organs. The kidneys are one of the first organs to be affected by decreased perfusion and are a significant clinical finding to indicate there is decreased perfusion to the body and organs.	**R**eport Urine Output < 30 mL/hr or trending ↓. Daily weights and compare.
Fluids are necessary for perfusion, but must be monitored closely, particularly when the decrease in perfusion is due to decreased pump action or failure. If there is excess fluid in the circulatory system, this causes an increased workload on the heart to pump the additional fluid. Diuretics are commonly used to reduce the volume the heart has to pump.	**F**luids: monitor amount, maintain patent IV line. (Note: ↓ fluids if HF or Cardiogenic Shock.)
Use "CLUSTER" *(Refer to Activity Tolerance later in this chapter)* to manage energy conservation with clients that have pump failure, infections, and/or inflammation of the heart. Prioritizing activities and pacing them with rest helps avoid an increased workload on the heart that results in decreased perfusion and inadequate oxygenation that can also lead to pain from ischemia.	**U**se "CLUSTER" to manage energy conservation *(Refer to Activity Tolerance in this chapter)*.
Support stockings or intermittent-compression devices help increase the return of blood to the heart when the heart is unable to adequately perfuse or if there is peripheral constriction or blockages that prevent adequate return of blood to the heart.	**S**upport stockings or intermittent-compression devices (except for DVT on affected leg).
Encourage ambulation/ROM is important to help increase perfusion and circulation. Monitoring the client's response to the activity (i.e., VS, report of pain, O₂ sat, etc.) will help determine if the client is able to tolerate the activity.	**E**ncourage ambulation/ROM ↑ perfusion/ circulation (except if there is chest pain, an infection of the heart, severe heart failure, or cardiomyopathy that requires rest).

(Manning, L. & Zager, L. (2014). Medical surgical nursing concepts made insanely easy!
A new approach to prioritization, Duluth, GA: ICAN Publishing, Inc., p. 164.)

APPENDIX D

Chapter 5

SAFETY SUMMARY: CONCEPT CARDIAC/PERIPHERAL PERFUSION

SYSTEM-SPECIFIC ASSESSMENT "PUMPS"	FIRST-DO PRIORITY INTERVENTIONS "PERFUSE"	EVALUATION OF EXPECTED OUTCOMES "PUMPS"
Pulses (peripheral & JVD) assess bilaterally & compare, capillary refill > 3 seconds, auscultate heart sounds (note presence of S_3 or S_4), heart rate, rhythm (pulse ↓ or ↑ with arrhythmias), & BP. Assess for ↓ level of consciousness (LOC), syncope.	**P**osition HOB ↑. NOTE: if BP decreases, lower HOB to semi-Fowler's or supine position (*Refer to PVD for specifics on positioning*). Give supplement O_2 as needed. Avoid restrictive clothes, cold, and nicotine.	**P**ulses and BP WDL for client
Urine output, (< 30 mL/hour), evaluate daily weights and compare.	**E**valuate VS and pulses (compare R & L), edema (compare R & L), lung sounds, ECG, CVP & hemodynamic monitoring. Evaluate surgical incision site for bleeding, circulation, skin temp, color, signs of infection, and healing.	**U**rine > 30 mL/hour
Moist lung sounds (adventitious) ↑ Resp, edema (compare R & L extremities).	**R**eport urine output < 30 mL/hour or trending ↓ , daily weights and compare.	**M**oist lung sounds resolved, no edema; respiratory rate WDL
Pain will vary (*Refer to Angina, MI, PVD for specifics*). Assess to see if pain increases with activity.	**F**luids: monitor amount, maintain patent IV line. Note: ↓ fluids if heart failure or cardiogenic shock.	**P**ain, none or managed
Skin color pale, cool extremities, ↑ temp (for infections of the heart or heart valves disorders).	**U**se "CLUSTER" to manage energy conservation (*Refer to Activity Tolerance in this chapter for specifics*).	**S**kin warm and dry, color WDL for client
	Support stockings or intermittent-compression devices (except for DVT on affected leg).	
	Encourage ambulation/ROM to increase perfusion and circulation (except if there is chest pain, an infection of the heart, severe heart failure, or cardiomyopathy that requires rest).	

(Manning, L. & Zager, L. (2014). Medical surgical nursing concepts made insanely easy! A new approach to prioritization, Duluth, GA: ICAN Publishing, Inc., p. 165.)

THE PATHOPHYSIOLOGY BEHIND ALTERATIONS IN OXYGENATION

OXYGENATION						
Obstruction	**Infection**	**Collapsed Lung**	**Pulmonary Artery Obstruction**	**Failure**	**Transport**	**Perfusion**
• Asthma • COPD (Emphysema Bronchitis) • Cystic Fibrosis	**Upper Respiratory Tract:** • Croup • Epiglottitis • Tonsillitis **Lower Respiratory Tract:** • Pneumonia • Tuberculosis • Severe Acute Respiratory Syndrome (SARS)	• Pneumo-thorax • Hemothorax • Tension pneumo-thorax	• Pulmonary Emboli	• Acute Respiratory Failure (ARF) • Acute Respiratory Distress Syndrome (ARDS)	**Anemia Issues:** • Aplastic • Folic Acid Deficiency • Iron Deficiency • Hemolytic • Pernicious • Thalassemia • Sickle Cell Anemia	*Refer to Concept Perfusion and Shock Chapter* • Aneurysm • Heart Failure • Peripheral Artery Disease • Shock

(Manning, L. & Zager, L. (2014). Medical surgical nursing concepts made insanely easy! A new approach to prioritization, Duluth, GA: ICAN Publishing, Inc., p. 124.)

LINKING PATHOPHYSIOLOGY TO
SYSTEM-SPECIFIC ASSESSMENTS FOR ALTERED OXYGENATION

PATHOPHYSIOLOGY	SYSTEM-SPECIFIC ASSESSMENTS "DYSPNEA"
Dyspnea may occur as a result of narrowed airways from bronchoconstriction (i.e., asthma) or obstruction (i.e., chronic bronchitis, cystic fibrosis); poor gas exchange in the alveoli, (i.e., pneumonia, pulmonary edema); impaired nerve function or inadequate muscle to assist with air movement into the lungs, (i.e., cervical spinal cord injury). Altered oxygen transport, such as with anemia, can result in dyspnea due to insufficient blood cells carrying oxygen. Altered perfusion as a result of a reduction in cardiac output, such as in a myocardial infarction, can result in dyspnea due to hypoxia. Orthopnea refers to an abnormal condition during which a client must sit or stand to breathe. Clients with COPD may prefer to sleep while leaning forward over a table.	**D**yspnea, orthopnea and nocturnal– assess.
Yes, vital signs will be elevated due to a physiological response to compensate for the decrease in oxygenation. Temperature may be increased due to an infection. The change in the respiratory rate is due to the increase work to breathe. If client is using pursed-lip breathing on exhalation, it is to assist in keeping airways open longer. Tachycardia may occur due to anxiety from not being able to breathe or from anemia. The pale skin and mucous membranes can be from anemia or hypoxemia. A late sign of hypoxemia is cyanosis. As the hypoxia increases, there can be a decrease in the perfusion of blood to the brain, resulting in a decrease in the LOC. *Geriatric clients will typically present with an acute confusion due to the lack of oxygen.*	**Y**es, early signs: ($\uparrow$ T, $\uparrow$ RR, $\uparrow$ HR, $\uparrow$ BP); restlessness; skin & mucous membranes pale; late signs: VS $\downarrow$, cyanosis, $\downarrow$ level of consciousness (LOC), lethargy, lightheadedness. (*Geriatric clients: acute confusion is early sign.*)
Secretions can change from clear to yellow in color, which may indicate an infection. Pink-tinged secretions that are thin and frothy are seen in pulmonary edema. These secretions are thin because it is combined with water. If the hydrostatic pressure is very high, small capillaries break and sputum becomes pink tinged.	**S**ecretions altered, productive cough (color, consistency, tenacity and odor). Pulmonary edema: pink-tinged, frothy sputum. Signs of infection (i.e., $\uparrow$ temp, $\uparrow$ WBC, yellow secretions).
Precipitating factors must be determined in order to develop an appropriate plan of action. For example if hypoxia is from a post-op respiratory infection, the priority of care is T, C, and DB; if it is from stress, the care is to assist with healthy coping mechanisms.	**P**recipitating factors: infection, immobility, allergens, stress, trauma, post-op complications, pleurisy.
Noting characteristics of the cough will assist in plan of care. The cough is a defensive attempt to expectorate secretions or extra fluid in the lungs.	**N**ote characteristics of the cough (i.e., dry, moist, productive), alleviating or aggravating factors, discomfort with breathing; symptoms with cough such a fever or shortness of breath).
Evaluate SaO$_2$ pulse oximetry readings are typically less than the defined limits due to the decrease in the oxygen available for perfusion. ABGs may reveal a respiratory acidosis due to hypoventilation, an increase in carbon dioxide (i.e., COPD). If client is hyperventilating, outcome would be respiratory alkalosis (i.e., anxiety). (*Refer to Concept Acid Base Balance chapter for specifics.*)	**E**valuate SaO$_2$ < 95% on arterial blood gases (ABGs), pulse oximetry < 92%.
Adventitious breath sounds may occur from the mucus or secretions in the bronchi.	**A**dventitious breath sounds (wheezes, crackles, atelectasis after post-op); immobility; arrhythmias; use of accessory muscles, asymmetrical chest expansion; activity intolerance.

(Manning, L. & Zager, L. (2014). Medical surgical nursing concepts made insanely easy! A new approach to prioritization, Duluth, GA: ICAN Publishing, Inc., p. 125.)

LINKING PATHOPHYSIOLOGY TO
FIRST-DO PRIORITY INTERVENTIONS FOR ALTERED OXYGENATION

PATHOPHYSIOLOGY	FIRST-DO PRIORITY INTERVENTIONS "BREATHE"
Breath sounds need to be assessed due to the potential alteration in air exchange from secretions, adventitious sounds from fluid and/or secretions; absent sounds due to a pneumothorax; or distant from COPD. Due to altered oxygenation, the client may experience some lightheadedness when upright. Oxygen supplement will assist with the hypoxia.	**B**reath sounds, SaO_2, vital signs, DYSPNEA assess and monitor; O_2 as needed, assess for arrhythmias; lightheadedness.
Reposition client sitting up due to the impaired gas exchange to assist with lung expansion. Clients with acute or chronic impaired oxygenation breathe more easily in high Fowler's position or semi-Fowler's position. These positions will facilitate the movement of the diaphragm away from the lungs which will decrease the workload of breathing.	**R**eposition to facilitate ventilation and perfusion, (i.e., HOB ↑, up in chair, ambulate, particularly after surgery).
Evaluation of the airway status is an ongoing priority of care for clients with alteration in oxygenation in order to know how to further intervene. In addition to the assessment, it is imperative to evaluate the functioning of the emergency equipment to assure it is working effectively in case the client needs assistance with mechanical ventilation. Clients may require intubation with either an endotracheal tube or tracheostomy tube. Humidified oxygen is delivered to the trachea and bronchi. If breathing support is needed, then the ventilator will control the RR and volume.	**E**valuate airway status; prepare for oxygen supplement, (i.e., ambu bag); initiate EMERGENCY management as needed, (i.e., CPR , mechanical ventilation).
Assess and document ABG values. ABGs may reveal a respiratory acidosis due to hypoventilation, an increase in carbon dioxide (i.e., COPD). If client is hyperventilating, outcome would be respiratory alkalosis (i.e., anxiety). (*Refer to Concept Acid Base Balance chapter for specifics.*) The color of the secretions will change from clear to yellow in color indicating an infection. The thin, pink-tinged secretions (because it is combined with water) are frothy and are seen with pulmonary edema. If the hydrostatic pressure is very high, small capillaries break and sputum becomes pink tinged. Oral care will minimize sores and dryness.	**A**ssess and document ABG values, sputum color, consistency and amount, good oral care every 2 hours.
The airway needs ongoing suctioning to remove the secretions in order to optimize airway patency. Chest physiotherapy and postural drainage are performed to loosen and move secretions into the large airways where they can be expectorated. Postural drainage uses gravity and different positions to remove secretions after they are loosened from specific lung segments.	**T**he airway needs to be suctioned PRN to maintain patency. Chest physiotherapy and postural drainage per protocol, bronchodilators and hand held nebulizers as prescribed.
Hand washing is a major nursing activity to prevent respiratory tract infections. If client does have a respiratory tract infection, then the PPE used will be based on the organism the client has (*Refer to Concept Infection Control chapter for specifics*). If there is an order for any type of cultures and to start antibiotics, obtain CULTURES 1st and then start the ANTIBIOTICS. *Doorknobs and countertops should be cleaned to prevent transmission of infections.*	**H**and washing, wear appropriate PPE, apply infection control standards (*i.e., room placement, assignment, etc.*); cultures, (before antibiotics, etc.).
Encourage deep breathing and coughing for clients (i.e., immobilized, pneumonia, COPD, etc.) will increase lung expansion and facilitate oxygen exchange. Fluids, based on medical condition, will liquefy secretions. Educate regarding coughing or sneezing into a tissue will decrease the particles dispersed into the air. Health Promotion is always important for compliance!	**E**ncourage deep breathing and coughing, incentive spirometer, evaluate outcome of medications. Educate/emotional support, encourage fluids based on clinical presentation.

(Manning, L. & Zager, L. (2014). Medical surgical nursing concepts made insanely easy! A new approach to prioritization, Duluth, GA: ICAN Publishing, Inc., p. 130.)

APPENDIX H

SAFETY SUMMARY: CONCEPT OXYGENATION

SYSTEM-SPECIFIC ASSESSMENT "DYSPNEA"	FIRST-DO PRIORITY INTERVENTIONS "BREATHE"	EVALUATION OF EXPECTED OUTCOMES "NO DYSPNEA"
Dyspnea, orthopnea & nocturnal	**B**reath sounds, SaO_2, vital signs, DYSPNEA assess & monitor; O_2 as needed, assess for arrhythmias; lightheadedness.	**D**yspnea, orthopnea & nocturnal NONE
Yes, early signs: ($\uparrow$ T, $\uparrow$ RR, $\uparrow$ HR, $\uparrow$ BP); restlessness; skin & mucous membranes pale; late signs: vital signs $\downarrow$, cyanosis, $\downarrow$ level of consciousness (LOC), lethargy, lightheadedness. (*Geriatric clients: acute confusion is early sign.*)	**R**eposition to facilitate ventilation & perfusion, (i.e., HOB $\uparrow$, up in chair, ambulate, particularly after surgery).	**Y**es, vital signs Normal, No restlessness, color pink; no lightheadedness
	Evaluate airway status; prepare for oxygen supplement, (i.e. ambu bag); initiate EMERGENCY management as needed, (i.e., CPR, mechanical ventilation).	**S**ecretions, sputum color clear
Secretions altered, productive cough (color, consistency, tenacity and odor). Pulmonary edema: pink-tinged, frothy sputum. Signs of infection (i.e., $\uparrow$ temp, $\uparrow$ WBC, yellow secretion, etc.).		**P**recipitating factors NONE
		NO cough
Precipitating factors: infection, immobility, allergens, stress, trauma, post op complications, pleurisy.	**A**ssess and document ABG values, sputum color, consistency & amount, good oral care every 2 hours.	**E**valuation of $SaO_2 > 95\%$ on arterial blood gases (ABGs), O_2 sat $> 92\%$
Note characteristics of the cough (i.e., dry, moist, productive), alleviating or aggravating factors, discomfort with breathing; symptoms with cough such a fever or shortness of breath).	**T**he airway needs to be suctioned PRN to maintain patency. Chest physiotherapy & postural drainage per protocol, bronchodilators & hand held nebulizers as prescribed.	**A**dventitious breath sounds, NONE; NO arrhythmias; NO use of accessory muscles; symmetrical chest expansion
	Hand washing, wear appropriate PPE, apply infection control standards (i.e., room placement, assignment, etc.); obtain cultures before antibiotics.	**N**O activity intolerance
Evaluate $SaO_2 < 95\%$ on arterial blood gases (ABGs), pulse oximetry $< 92\%$.		
Adventitious breath sounds (wheezes, crackles, atelectasis after post-op); immobility; arrhythmias; use of accessory muscles, asymmetrical chest expansion; activity intolerance.	**E**ncourage deep breathing & coughing, incentive spirometer, evaluate outcome of medications. **E**ducate/emotional support, encourage fluids based on clinical presentation.	

(Manning, L. & Zager, L. (2014). Medical surgical nursing concepts made insanely easy! A new approach to prioritization, Duluth, GA: ICAN Publishing, Inc., p. 131.)

ENGAGING THE LEARNER ACTIVITIES

INDEPENDENT STUDENT REFLECTIVE EXERCISE
LINKED TO PROFESSIONAL AND NCLEX® STANDARDS

RESOURCES NEEDED FOR ACTIVITY	*The Eight Step Approach for Student Clinical Success* (Zager, Manning & Herman, 2018)
Standards	**Student Instructions**
Physiological Integrity: Physiological Adaptation Perform focused assessment (system-specific assessment). Identify pathophysiology related to an acute or chronic condition. Evaluate the effectiveness of the treatment regimen for a client with an acute/chronic diagnosis.	**Based on what you read in this chapter, answer the following reflective questions.** *(Refer to the Appendices in this chapter)* 1. What system-specific assessment findings are associated with the concept of decreased cardiac perfusion? 2. What pathophysiology was connected to the first-do priority interventions for decreased cardiac perfusion? 3. Based on the analysis of the assessments, what evaluation data would indicate the expected outcomes have been met for cardiac perfusion? 4. What is the pathophysiological explanation for the first-do priority intervention of elevating the head of the bed for a client with alteration in oxygenation? 5. What are the possible pathophysiological explanations for why decreased cardiac perfusion is related to an alteration in oxygenation?

NOTES

Preparing for Successful Simulation

Kate K. Chappell, MSN, APRN, CPNP-PC

IN THIS CHAPTER YOU WILL LEARN HOW TO:

➤ Prepare for simulation

➤ Participate in simulation

➤ Receive and participate in debriefing

INTRODUCTION

Simulation is an important part of your nursing education. "Simulation education is a bridge between classroom learning and real-life clinical experience" (Simulation for Society in Healthcare, 2016). You will be able to perform aspects of client care in a safe environment for you to learn, make mistakes without risk to the client, receive feedback, and perform the care again to reinforce your learning (Simulation for Society in Healthcare).

The International Nursing Association for Clinical Simulation and Learning (INACSL) has developed Standards of Best Practice: Simulation[SM] to promote consistency and quality across nursing programs using simulation so it benefits students in the way that it was intended. Simulation is an excellent opportunity to solidify your technical and thinking skills. Simulation also prepares you for challenges you will encounter in clinical practice after graduation. These skills include, communicating with others on the healthcare team, recognizing trends in patient data, and evaluating progress in time-sensitive situations.

You may encounter different types of manikins in your simulation lab. There are four different types of manikins:

✦ **High Fidelity**— "Experiences using full scale computerized patient simulators, virtual reality or standardized patients that are extremely realistic and provide a high level of interactivity and realism for the learner" (NLN-SIRC, 2013, p. S-6).

+ **Moderate or Mid-Fidelity**—"Experiences that are more technologically sophisticated such as computer-based self-directed learning systems simulations in which the participant relies on a two-dimensional focused experience to problem solve, perform a skill, and make decisions" (NLN-SIRC, 2013, p. S-7). *Mid-Fidelity* can also be used to describe the use of manikins "more realistic than static low fidelity ones having breath sounds, heart sounds and/or pulses" (NLN-SIRC).

+ **Low Fidelity**—"Experiences such as case studies, role-playing, using partial task trainers or static manikins to immerse students in a clinical situation or practice a specific skill" (NLN-SIRC, 2013, p. S-7).

+ **Task Trainers**—"Simulators that are used to practice a skill such as an IV arm that is used to practice IV insertions skills" (Kardong-Edgren, et al., 2011, p. S4–S5).

The information and tools in this chapter will give you the strategies you need to be Successful in Simulation!

PREPARE FOR SIMULATION

Preparing for simulation is as important as preparing for clinical in the live patient healthcare setting. Orientation may be done through an online course management system (i.e., Blackboard), conducted in the simulation lab, or a combination of the two.

Common topics in an orientation will include:

+ Simulation lab layout.

+ Manikins that will be used that may be different from other manikins you may have used to include the sounds and functions.

+ Medication dispensing machine.

+ Available equipment and supplies.

Please refer to **Helpful Tips When Doing Simulation** (Appendix A) for additional guidance for preparation.

Simulation may be graded or non-graded and may be referred to as high-stakes or low-stakes simulation. As part of your preparation, you need to know if you will be graded during the simulation and what the objectives and the purpose of the simulation activity are. The focus in low-stakes simulation is to reinforce your learning. The focus on high-stakes simulation is to assess your competency. The definitions of low and high-stakes simulation are:

+ **Low-stakes simulation** is ungraded and used primarily for learning experiences. It provides constructive feedback for you to be able to improve (NLN-SIRC, 2013).

+ **High-stakes simulation** is used for evaluation of your readiness or competence for course-specific skills or content, or to determine if you need clinical skills remediation (Meakim, Boese, Decker, Franklin, Gloe, Lioce, Sando, & Borum, 2013).

Simulation can sometimes feel very challenging whether it is graded or not. Students often report feeling "on the spot" and that it is harder to perform well in simulation than in a live clinical setting. It is undeniable, you ARE more "on the spot" in simulation than live clinical—you are performing care independently in a way that isn't possible in clinical. But, how you approach simulation can influence how successful you are in simulation! The list below gives you strategies to help you put your best foot forward.

- **Treat the manikins as if they are a real person.** Help your brain "believe" this is a real situation and your thinking and actions will come more naturally!

  - Talk to the client as you normally would during your assessment and care. The verbal exchange with your client will give you additional information about your client's anxiety level, if they get short of breath while talking, etc.

  - Tell the client what you are going to do and ask for their part in participation (i.e., asking them to hold still while you start the IV, or hold their breath during a chest X-ray).

  - Do things "for real" to keep your brain focused on what is happening instead of thinking about what isn't real or what actions you can skip.

- **Prepare for simulation.** Plan ahead so you don't feel "caught off guard" or "behind" on the expectations before you start your activity!

  - Start off on a good foot by dressing appropriately, having the books or equipment you need with you, and being on time to the lab!

  - Use information your faculty provides about the client, the setting, and the expectations to help you get in the right mindset for the clinical experience.

- **Plan your approach to the simulation.**
  - What do you plan to do 1st, 2nd, and 3rd when you enter the room? What would be a possible complication or new finding that would change this plan? What would your first step be in that situation? Thinking ahead will help you stay calm and focused no matter what happens in the simulation.

- **Three simple rules** to keep you on track during a simulation or in a live clinical situation:
  - **Safety is the Number One Priority!** Make safety a priority in every action you take. The actions in the simulation room should be the same you would take on your first day working as an RN. If it is outside of the RN's scope of practice (i.e., administering a medication without an order or something you have never been taught such as inserting a tracheostomy on your own), it is probably NOT the right move.

  - **Practice within your scope of practice and seek help when appropriate.** If you have done everything the RN can/should do to manage the situation, it is time to get help or further information! Demonstrating you know how and when to seek help or others' expertise is essential for patient safety. Simulation is an excellent place to get that experience.

✦ **Use positive self-talk to stay on track.** Tell yourself, "I can do this; I do have the skills to take care of a client with this problem." Saying or thinking negatively that simulation makes you nervous reinforces that you should be nervous which can make you more nervous! Positive self-talk and thinking during simulation will help you control some of the triggers for stress. When your brain is in "fight-or-flight," it is difficult to critically think or reason about how to care for your client!

When you receive the information about your upcoming simulation experience, please prepare! Depending on your faculty's plan and the type of activity, you may receive information before the day of the activity or you may have only a brief preparation time before the simulation begins. Important areas in your preparation include:

✦ Review the information about the given client's diagnosis, (i.e., diabetes, heart failure, healthy newborn, etc.) and current situation (i.e., admission, shift assessment, home health visit, etc.).

✦ Review what to include in your system-specific assessments (i.e., lab values, procedure reports, etc.).

✦ Consider what might be the priority concepts based on the involved body system and the system-specific pathophysiology of the given medical diagnosis.

✦ Review potential priority interventions (i.e., medications, potential reactions, repositioning, monitoring lab values, additional vital signs or assessments, etc.).

✦ Review the expected outcomes for the priority concepts.

✦ Consider what the potential complications might be.

✦ Review the "RISKS" to the client (i.e., infection control, safety, equipment, etc.).

Preparing, by reviewing the above information, will help you anticipate the first actions needed in the simulation activity.

Simulation Preparation Tool (Appendix B), is a tool to help guide your preparation and thinking for simulation. Use the tool while you are reviewing the information listed above. If you do this, you will be mentally prepared for success! **The Example of How to Use the Simulation Preparation Tool** (Appendix C) shows how to use the tool to prepare before a simulation exercise after receiving your preparation information.

PARTICIPATE IN THE SIMULATION

Preparation ahead of time helps during the simulation just like it does when you are going to clinical. Usually, you will do the same things each time you enter the simulation room. Practice these actions until you have them memorized. Doing familiar actions will decrease anxiety. When you enter the simulation room:

✦ Introduce yourself.

✦ Perform handwashing.

✦ Note equipment, IVs, and other items attached to client.

✦ Talk to the client throughout the simulation.

✦ Note healthcare provider orders as appropriate.

✦ Review the medication administration record (MAR) and prepare medications as appropriate.

✦ Complete your system-specific assessment based on the client situation (i.e., VS, lab values, cardiac monitor, etc.).

✦ Respond to simulation client condition and changes (i.e., changes in VS, cardiac monitor, client verbal and/or manikin responses).

✦ Do priority interventions as appropriate.

✦ Evaluate the client's response to your interventions.

✦ Give an SBAR report as needed. (Refer to Chapter 2 in this book for Appendix F, **Example of SBAR Report For Patient Handoff At Change Of Shift;** Appendix G, **Preparing an SBAR For Call To Healthcare Provider;** and Appendix H, **Example of SBAR Format To Make A Call To The Healthcare Provider**).

✦ Document as appropriate for simulation.

REMEMBER to TALK OUT LOUD!!
Talk out loud during simulation so your faculty knows what you are trying to observe, assess, or do!

(Faculty may need the prompt to realize the manikin needs to speak, cough, or have an assessment change!)

RECEIVE AND PARTICIPATE IN DEBRIEFING

Debriefing from simulation is just like talking about a live clinical day. It is absolutely essential for you to learn. Debriefing reinforces the appropriate clinical decisions you made and illustrates what you did not know but need to know. Faculty will give you feedback to help with your learning process. Be open to it! Feedback should lead to self-reflection, part of clinical reasoning and the role of a professional nurse.

The debriefing experience will start with the following questions that you will reflect upon independently before the group does the debriefing discussion.

+ What is the first thing that comes to mind about the simulation experience?

+ What went well and why?

+ What would you do differently and why?

(Dreifuerst, 2009, 2012)

At the end of the debriefing, your clinical instructor will lead a discussion of the reflection points (DML) for the specific scenario with these three points:

+ Thinking-in-action (thinking that occurs during the simulation).

+ Thinking-on-action (thinking that occurs while reflecting after the simulation).

+ Thinking-beyond-action (thinking of how the experience will apply to future client's clinical situations).

(Dreifuerst, 2009, 2012)

Here is an example of the three reflection points with an emergency department (ED) client simulation. The goal of the scenario was to respond to a client with an increased heart rate and respiratory rate after a vehicle collision. Based on the assessment during the simulation, it was determined that the client had acute bleeding due to a "seatbelt" abdominal injury causing hypovolemic shock.

+ **Thinking-in-action**: What system-specific assessments based on the pathophysiology distinguish between airway obstruction, hypovolemia, and a panic attack?

+ **Thinking-on-action**: Given a client with hypovolemia from acute abdominal bleeding, what are the priority interventions?

+ **Thinking-beyond-action**: What potential complications will you assess for in future clients who have been in a motor vehicle collision? What questions can you ask about where they were located in the car to get more information about potential issues?

Simulation provides you with a wonderful opportunity to reinforce your clinical decision making in a safe environment. Each simulation experience will help maximize your learning and give you confidence as you successfully transition from a student nurse to a graduate nurse.

HELPFUL TIPS WHEN DOING SIMULATION

Required Equipment
- Stethoscope.
- Penlight.
- Scissors.
- Pen/paper (clipboard).
- Watch with second hand.

Professional Appearance
- Hair in compliance with clinical dress code.
- Proper uniform with name tag.
- Nails clean and short.
- Minimal jewelry.

Teamwork
- Work as a team-no one person is in charge unless specifically assigned by the faculty member.
- Prior to starting the scenario divide up activities that need to be done and change around from week to week (i.e., if student A does vital signs one week student B will do them the next).
- Each student should actively participate in checking orders, preparing meds, checking IV site and fluids, communicating with the client, etc.
- All assessments, observations, communications, and tasks should be communicated **out loud** to facilitate group decision making and give faculty insight into your thinking/planning process.
- If you feel you are on the right track or another student is about to perform an unsafe/inappropriate action, don't back down! Talk it out with your team.

Functional Points
- Healthcare Provider (HCP) orders and medication record are available at the bedside.
- Know where the supplies needed are kept for the scenario.
- Know the method for calling the HCP or other ancillary personnel.
- Lab results will be made available only if requested. If none are available the facilitator will state as much.
- **Treat the manikin as a real client** … ask them questions and respond to their comments and questions.

REMEMBER THAT ACTIVITIES YOU DO IN THE HOSPITAL WHEN ENTERING THE CLIENT'S ROOM ARE ALSO EXPECTATIONS DURING SIMULATION (i.e., handwashing, identify yourself using first and last name, your role as an RN, and identify your client using two identifiers).

Remember you signed a Confidentiality Agreement to maintain scenario integrity. Sharing information devalues student experiences, skews evaluation and/or grading expectations against earlier teams, and decreases learning experience for later teams.

Developed by Erin McKinney, MN, RN, RNC-O

APPENDIX B

SIMULATION PREPARATION TOOL
("SAFETY" TOOL ADAPTED FOR SIMULATION)

Simulation Scenario/Activity: _____

Setting: _____

Medical Diagnosis/Problem: _____

Goal: _____

	System/Medical Diagnosis/Problem	System/Medical Diagnosis/ Problem	System/Medical Diagnosis/ Problem
System-Specific Physiology			
System-Specific Assessments, Labs, Diagnostic Procedures			
Analyze Concept(s)	Concept	Concept	Concept
First-Do Priority Interventions; Medications			
Evaluation of Expected Outcomes			
Trend Potential Complications			
You Must Manage Care to Prevent "RISKS" to Clients			
Health Promotion and Discharge Planning			
Client Specific Planning	Other disciplines or departments consults needed? Specific safety needs? Specific infection control needs? Where to get additional information (i.e., family, last facility, or unit, etc.)? Coordination for transfer (i.e., to another unit, another facility, home, etc.)?		

"SAFETY" Tool (Manning, L. & Zager, L. (2014. p 7). Adapted by Kate K. Chappell, MSN, APRN, CPNP-PC

EXAMPLE OF HOW TO USE THE SIMULATION PREPARATION TOOL
(Use before a simulation, during pre-briefing, or before lab if information provided.)

Information provided by faculty: 74-year-old male with acute confusion admitted to the ED.

Simulation Scenario/Activity: 74-year-old male from long-term care facility with acute confusion
Setting: Emergency Department
Medical Diagnosis/Problem: Acute confusion
Goal: Prioritize assessments and plan of care

System-Specific Physiology	Concept Fluid and Electrolytes	Concept Intracranial Regulation (Neuro	Concept Infection
System-Specific Assessments, Labs, Diagnostic Procedures	• VS: HR–96 bpm, RR–18, BP–156/88, T–99.1°F • Pulse ox–96% on room air • Weight–166 lbs. • History of weight changes–none • Labs (electrolytes, BUN, Cr., urine osmolality, specific gravity, etc.–WDL) • Urine–dark, cloudy with strong odor • Recent meds, possible ingestions of other meds–none applicable	• Pupillary response–equal & reactive • Level of consciousness–lethargic and confused x 3 (day, time & orientation) • ROM, sensation–full ROM • Neuro checks–WDL • Possible bleed (CVA)–no history of hypertension, falls • CT scan results–none ordered • History of past confusion–none • Mini Mental Status Exam–WDL • No history of past mental health diagnoses or symptoms • Family reports client is normally active and mentally alert • Medications–not on any anticoagulants	• Temperature–99.1°F • WBC count–11,000mm^3 • Urine–dark, cloudy with strong odor • Recent past infections–history of UTIs
Analyze Concept(s)	• Fluid and Electrolyte Balance Altered (suspect client may be dehydrated)	• Impaired intracranial regulation (no system-specific assessments to confirm)	• Infection (based on labs and urine color and odor)
First-Do Priority Interventions; Medications	• Daily Weight • Monitor I & O • VS every 4 hours • Monitor lab results and report abnormalities to healthcare provider • Medications N/A	• Monitor neuro status every 4 hours, report and document changes • Medications N/A	• Monitor VS–document and evaluate trending • Strict I & O • Use standard precautions • Document color, odor of urine • Medications: administer antibiotics as ordered

cont'd on next page

APPENDIX C

EXAMPLE OF HOW TO USE THE SIMULATION PREPARATION TOOL *(cont'd)*
(Use before a simulation, during pre-brief, or before lab if information provided.)

System-Specific Physiology	Concept Fluid and Electrolytes	Concept Intracranial Regulation (Neuro	Concept Infection
Evaluation of Expected Outcomes	• Fluid Balance (i.e., I & O, lips and mucous membranes moist, etc.) • No weight loss > 2lbs/day • Labs WDL (i.e., serum sodium 139 mEq/L)	• Level of consciousness and orientation return to client's baseline	• WBC count WDL • Temperature WDL • VS stable • Urine clear, yellow
Trend Potential Complications	• Reassess VS (note changes trending up or down)	• Assess for increased confusion • Assess for new behaviors (combative, impulsive) that increase safety risk • Assess changes in pupils, ROM	• Increase in temperature • WBC count continues to rise • Urine remains dark, cloudy • Client reports pain on voiding, abdominal or flank pain
You Must Manage Care to Prevent "RISKS" to Clients	• Fall precautions (particularly if client incontinent or hurrying to bathroom, and/or continued confusion)	• Close supervision • Hide/cover, secure IV or O_2 lines • Check 2 methods of identification (name band, picture, etc.)	• Fall precautions (particularly if client incontinent or hurrying to bathroom, and/or continued confusion)
Health Promotion and Discharge Planning	• Risks for causative factors (i.e., dehydration, not drinking adequate fluids) • Encourage fluids • Follow up with primary care appointment	• If chronic or risk to recur, use alert button or other monitoring devices • Identification & health information on person always • Home safety • Family/Friends contacts	• Instruct client about preventing UTIs • Instruct client to report to healthcare provider early signs of infection
Client Specific Planning	**Other disciplines or departments consults needed?** (Long-term care facility) **Setting specific safety needs?** (Evaluate continually the need for fall precautions) **Setting specific infection control needs?** (Use standard precautions, minimize cross-contact between patients in close proximity, clean equipment between uses) **Possible last unit or location if need additional information?** (Information from the long-term care facility, friend/family who brought him in) **Possible next step up for transfer?** (Transfer to medical/surgical floor) **Possible next step down for transfer?** (Discharge back to long-term care facility)		

"SAFETY" Tool (Manning, L. & Zager, L. (2014. p 7). Adapted by Kate K. Chappell, MSN, APRN, CPNP-PC

ENGAGING THE LEARNER ACTIVITIES

STUDENT-CENTERED LEARNING ACTIVITIES
LINKED TO PROFESSIONAL AND NCLEX® STANDARDS

Resources Needed for Activities	*The Eight-Step Approach for Student Clinical Success* (Zager, Manning & Herman, 2018)
Standards	**Student Instructions**
Management of Care Organize workload to manage time effectively. Serve as a resource person to other staff.	**Scavenger Hunt for Simulation** 1. Work in groups of 2 or 3 to find where the items on the list are located in your simulation lab. a. When you are done, you and your fellow students will conduct a tour for your faculty to show them where the items are located in your simulation lab.

Safety & Infection Control
 	
Ensure proper identification of client when providing care. Apply principles of infection control (i.e., hand hygiene). Assure appropriate and safe use of equipment in performing client care.
	First Assessment of Client and Environment
	
	2. Practice in pairs the series of actions necessary when you enter a client's room in simulation and/or clinical for the first assessment of your client and their environment. Practice the actions prior to the simulation and /or clinical. Remind each other of the actions if necessary.
	
	  a. Knock on door before entering.
	
	  b. Greet the client and/or family members when you enter.
	
	  c. Introduce yourself.
	
	  d. Wash your hands.
	
	  e. Identify client by 2 methods.
	
	  f. Check provider orders.
	
	  g. Check the MAR.
	
	  h. Assess information provided on simulation monitor and equipment in the room (i.e., Foley, IV pump, drains, ambu bag for peds, etc.).
	
	  i. Perform a safety check (i.e., bedrails, bed in position, call light, etc.).
	
	  j. Talk out loud your actions, assessment findings, interventions, and the response of the client (manikin).

cont'd on next page

ENGAGING THE LEARNER ACTIVITIES

Chapter 6

STUDENT-CENTERED LEARNING ACTIVITIES
LINKED TO PROFESSIONAL AND NCLEX® STANDARDS *(cont'd)*

Resources Needed for Activities	*The Eight-Step Approach for Student Clinical Success* (Zager, Manning & Herman, 2018)
Standards	**Student Instructions**

Management of Care
 	
Organize workload to manage time effectively.
	Simulation Preparation Tool
	(Refer to Appendix B)
	
	1. Complete the **Simulation Preparation Tool** (Appendix B) on the assigned client scenario prior to simulation.
	
	  a. During debriefing, identify any information you needed that was missing on your Simulation Preparation Tool.
	
	  b. Refer to **Example of How to Use the Simulation Preparation Tool** (Appendix C) for reference.

Safety & Infection Control
 	
Protect client from injury (i.e., falls, electrical hazards). Follow institution's policy regarding restraints and safety devices.
	Safety—What Is Wrong With This Room?
	
	2. Determine what is wrong in the room for an elderly client on suicide precautions.
	
	  a. List the safety concerns for the client based on age and clinical conditions.
	
	  b. Determine corrective actions.

CHAPTER 7

Evaluating Clinical Performance

IN THIS CHAPTER YOU WILL LEARN ABOUT:

- Criteria for clinical evaluation
- Using feedback effectively
- Participating in the evaluation process

One of the most anxiety-producing aspects of being a student is the clinical evaluation process. Your clinical instructor has the responsibility of evaluating whether you are able to give safe and effective care at your current level and are prepared to move forward to the next semester or to graduation. In this chapter, we will describe the process of clinical evaluation.

Evaluation is the ongoing process of observing, measuring, and judging your progress toward achievement of clinical performance outcomes. You need to know what evaluation criteria will be used and what the consequences will be if you do not meet the criteria (Koharchnik, Weideman, Walters, & Hardy, 2015). Effective evaluation will:

- Improve your skills and abilities.
- Motivate your development.
- Achieve learning outcomes.

CRITERIA FOR CLINICAL EVALUATION

Faculty determine expectations and clinical outcomes based on established standards of practice and patient safety. In your course syllabus, you will find the expected student clinical outcomes with clear measurable evaluation criteria. There are two areas of clinical evaluation, safe and effective clinical practice and profession behavior that you will be held accountable for.

Your syllabus will define what constitutes unsafe care practices. These will include but are not limited to:

✦ Failure to follow the 7 Rights of Medication Administration.

✦ Number and nature of medication errors allowed as part of the learning process.

✦ Failure to follow infection control standards.

✦ Failure to follow patient safety standards.

✦ Failure to adhere to HIPAA laws.

✦ Failure to communicate important clinical information to the clinical instructor or nursing staff during and at the end of shift.

✦ Failure to document nursing assessments, interventions, and evaluation of care.

✦ Performing nursing actions without supervision when supervision is required.

✦ Action or event that could result in harm or death of a client.

Criteria will also include expectations for attendance, tardiness, and professional behaviors. Other clinical expectations as outlined in Chapter 2 also serve as guidelines for evaluation.

USING FEEDBACK EFFECTIVELY

Timely feedback is necessary for learning (Koharchnik, Weideman, Walters, & Hardy, 2015). Feedback provides information on your strengths and weaknesses. The more timely the feedback, the more powerful it is. Feedback helps to clearly define the expectations on what you need to do each week to meet the clinical learning outcomes.

The fear of receiving feedback in clinical is shared by many students. It is difficult to hear negative feedback about your clinical performance. Always remember that feedback is an important part of the learning experience. What you may perceive as negative feedback from your clinical instructor, is constructive feedback intended to help you improve your clinical performance. Avoid being defensive and be open to the information your clinical instructor is giving you. Reflect on the feedback, ask questions for clarification, and develop a plan for improvement.

The following "Pitfalls" illustrate what NOT to do when receiving performance evaluation feedback from your clinical instructor:

✦ Avoid feedback.
  Pitfall: You will have no idea how you are doing.

✦ Avoid negative body language.
   Pitfall: Rolling your eyes and sighing are disrespectful and convey a negative attitude.

✦ Avoid the snapback.
   Pitfall: Responding defensively without thinking closes your mind to constructive feedback.

Other ineffective and unacceptable responses to feedback include:

✦ Expressing yourself in highly emotional terms.

✦ Making dire predictions like, "I might as well just quit nursing school" or "I am never going to pass this clinical."

✦ Making statements such as, "I never have had trouble with a clinical instructor before you."

Here are two examples of a student failing to meet the expectation of being prepared for clinical. Read the examples and ask yourself, which student do I want to be?

> **Example 1:**
>
> A student comes unprepared to clinical and states, "I was unable to find the information about my medications I am to administer today."

> **Example 2:**
>
> A student comes unprepared to clinical and states, "I was unable to find the information on my medications I am to administer today. I looked in my medication book and searched the web. This morning I plan to call pharmacy to get the information on the medications."

In the first example, the student failed to meet the clinical expectation of being prepared and to provide a safe care environment for the client.

We hope you chose the second example. This time the student took the initiative to meet the requirements for being prepared for clinical. The student's action represents information searching and problem solving, both excellent clinical reasoning attributes.

PARTICIPATING IN THE EVALUATION PROCESS

The concept map provides a valuable tool for you to use in clinical and provides your clinical instructor information about your thinking. The most important aspects of the concept map are that you can see the progression of your thinking and the development of your clinical judgment. The concept map is an evolving document that changes as the client's condition changes and as you improve your ability to provide appropriate care and make clinical decisions in both clinical and in simulation. **Preparing for Clinical Using the "SAFETY" Model** (Appendix A) and **Helpful Tips When Doing Simulation** (Refer to Chapter 6, Appendix A) will help you be prepared for both clinical and simulation.

Below are ways your clinical instructor may use the concept map as an evaluation tool.

✦ The initial concept map you prepare before beginning clinical assures your instructor that you are prepared to implement appropriate care for your client.

✦ You will be evaluated on your ability to make changes based on your assessment of the client, the client's response to the care, and evaluation and judgment about the care given.

Your clinical instructor knows you are becoming more sophisticated in your clinical reasoning when you are able to evaluate and use clinical judgment to make decisions about what care is needed in the future. An example of the criteria that can be used to grade the concept map can be found in Chapter 4, **Rubric Grading Tool for Adult Health Concept Map Example** (Appendix B).

As we stated earlier, evaluation is an ongoing process. Clinical instructors are looking for trends in your clinical performance. Weekly clinical evaluations are done to give you timely feedback about your progress, what you are doing well, and what you need to improve.

The purpose of the evaluation tool is to define the clinical outcomes the faculty have determined are necessary to meet clinical objectives. The evaluation criteria measure what you are expected to achieve. The **Example Evaluation Tool** (Appendix B) reflects criteria that you might be evaluated on (i.e., the nursing process, patient safety standards, clinical application of key NCLEX® standards, professional behaviors, and required written clinical care plans or concept maps, etc.) The course syllabus will state the process for clinical evaluation to include when counseling is necessary, what constitutes a clinical day failure, and when the clinical day failures result in course failure.

As you review the example evaluation tool, ask yourself, "What can I do to demonstrate what I am learning to my clinical instructor?" This is a great question considering that most of the time there is one clinical instructor and at least 8 students! Here are some suggestions:

✦ Wow your instructor by being prepared. (Refer to **Preparing for Clinical Using the "SAFETY" Model**, Appendix A).

✦ Keep your clinical instructor and your nurse informed about what you are doing.

✦ Impress your clinical instructor with needed changes you made in the care of your client based on your assessments.

✦ Demonstrate you know how to give an SBAR report *(Refer to Chapter 2, Appendix D).*

✦ Write about what you have learned in your reflection paper or journal.

✦ Share your contributions in post-conference.

✦ Take the initiative to find new learning experiences.

Weekly evaluation provides you the necessary information about your progress. As a student, you probably do not like to receive a "Needs Improvement." This does not indicate failure. It alerts you that there is a need for additional work in this area. It becomes unsatisfactory if week by week you are not making improvements in the same area. Remember, you are a student and you will need improvement! If your clinical performance does not improve, your clinical instructor may decide a counseling session is needed to outline performance improvement criteria.

A counseling session serves to notify you formally that your performance is unsatisfactory. There are two levels of counseling that your instructor may use:

✦ The counseling session identifies needed actions or behaviors to progress and includes consequences if you do not improve.

✦ The counseling session identifies a significant event or action that resulted in, or potentially could have resulted in, client harm. It includes the consequences (i.e., clinical day failure or course failure).

It does not matter when an unsafe event occurs. If it was unsafe on your first day of clinical, it is unsafe on your last day of clinical. A common structure for counseling is the "**STAR**" format (Refer to **STAR Counseling Form**, Appendix C). This is a concise format that keeps both you and your clinical instructor focused on the facts of the situation.

STAR FORMAT FOR COUNSELING

S Situation: Describe the situation

T Task: What was supposed to be accomplished, or what were the requirements, standards of practice or policies that were not met? Include standards or policies as appropriate.

A Action: Plan for Action: What do I need to do to improve?

Consequences: What are the consequences if you do not correct your performance? A time frame for improvement must be stated.

R Results: Follow-up sessions: Were actions accomplished? What was the outcome?

If it is decided that a counseling session is necessary, here is what may occur:

✦ You will be informed that your clinical instructor is concerned about your clinical performance and you will be notified when the counseling session will occur.

✦ A counseling form such as the "STAR" format will describe the situation with specific information.

✦ Most likely the course coordinator or other neutral party will witness the counseling session.

✦ You will be notified of the scheduled counseling time.

✦ The structure of the counseling session will include the purpose of the meeting, introduction of the witness, and begin with discussion of the situation as written on the counseling form.

✦ You need to be prepared to stay on the topic that is being discussed. Now is not the time to bring up other issues.

✦ Although it may be very difficult, try not to become emotional. Ask for a moment to excuse yourself if you need to control your emotions.

✦ After the clinical instructor has presented the situation, you will be given an opportunity to express your side of the story. There is usually a place on the form for you to write your comments.

✦ After you present your side of the story, the clinical instructor will discuss the actions you must take to be satisfactory and the consequences if satisfactory performance is not met.

✦ At the conclusion of the session, you will be asked to sign the form. Your signature only indicates you have seen the form and the session occurred. You can write in the comment section if you disagree.

✦ You will be given a copy of the counseling statement (Refer to **Example STAR Counseling Form**, Appendix D).

✦ REMAIN CALM AT ALL TIMES!!!!!!

Most of the time, the evaluation process is a positive experience. Remind yourself that the evaluation process is to help improve your skills and abilities, motivate you for future growth, and best of all, be successful in achieving clinical learning outcomes.

STUDYING WITH THE "SAFETY" MODEL

S	A	F	E	T	Y
System-Specific Physiology Assessments Labs/Procedures	**Analysis of Concepts**	**First-Do Priority Interventions**	**Evaluation of Expected Outcomes**	**Trend Potential Complications**	**You Must Manage Care to Prevent "RISK" to Clients**
Identify the pathophysiology related to the client's condition. Based on the focused assessment, what vital sign changes require a response? What are the signs and symptoms that require intervention and indicate potential complications? What lab values and diagnostic tests require follow-up or intervention?	What are the priority concepts based on the assessment of the client?	What are the priority interventions based on the system-specific assessments for the concepts identified? Which clients should be seen first or what interventions should be done first based on the assessment findings? What medications are ordered for administration and is there a priority based on the client's presenting clinical findings (i.e., serum glucose results, complaint of pain, etc.)?	Was the desired outcome for the client met (i.e., did the bleeding stop, did the breath sounds improve, did vital signs return to within the desired limits for the client, etc.)? Was the therapeutic effect of the administered medications achieved? Are there additional interventions required to meet the expected outcomes?	What are the trends and changes in the client's condition that require intervention? What are the priority interventions needed to prevent complications or prevent further complications? What system-specific assessments require ongoing contrasting, comparing, and trending?	Are the orders accurate and appropriate for this client? What "**RISK**" does the client have? *(Refer to "RISK" in this chapter)*

Questions based on the National Council of State Boards of Nursing, Inc. NCLEX-RN® Test Plan Activities, 2018.

"SAFETY" Model copyrighted by I CAN Publishing®, Inc., 2007. Questions adapted from (Manning & Zager, 2014, p 6).

APPENDIX B

Chapter 7

CLINICAL EVALUATION TOOL

Clinical Evaluation Tool Using "SAFETY" Model

Student Name:		Mid-Term				Final			
Clinical Date:									
PERFORMANCE OUTCOMES	S	NI	U	NA	S	NI	U	NA	

(Evaluation columns repeated: S / NI / U for multiple clinical dates, with Mid-Term and Final sections)

Performance Outcomes				
Prepared for all facets of clinical day, (care based on SAFETY (i.e., patho, asses, labs, diag tests, interventions, skills, meds, etc).				
System-Specific Assessment				
Performs system-specific assessments based on pathophysiology of disease & client need; reports/documents, assessments.				
Reports/documents clinical findings; Recognizes deviations from client's normal.				
Reviews & reports lab/diagnostic test findings that deviate from normal.				
Analysis: Concepts/ Outcomes				
Analysis of concepts, expected outcomes appropriate & measureable based on assessment findings.				
Idenitifies if client condition is acute/chronic.				
First-Do Priority Interventions				
Plans & prioritizes delivery of care/orders (interventions).				
Perform/document invasive nursing procedures with supervision only.				
Sterile procedure/ standard of care followed.				
Medication protocol/preparation/administration/ documentation (i.e., *Checks MAR against orders *Prepares/calculates dosage appropriately *Has needed data (i.e., VS, labs, etc.).				

Page 1

CLINICAL EVALUATION TOOL (cont'd)

Student Name: _____

Clinical Evaluation Tool Using "SAFETY" Model

Clinical Date:	S	NI	U	S	NI	U	S	NI	U	S	NI	U	S	NI	U	S	NI	U	Mid-Term S	NI	U	NA	S	NI	U	S	NI	U	S	NI	U	S	NI	U	S	NI	U	Final S	NI	U	NA
PERFORMANCE OUTCOMES																																								
Identifies client x 2 with every medication administered.																																								
Administers medications under supervision of instructor; Never administer, Sub cu, IV, IM, nasal gastric, peg without instructor.																																								
Evaluation of Expected Outcomes																																								
Evaluation of progress toward expected outcomes.																																								
Makes changes in plan of care as appropriate.																																								
Evaluates medications for expected outcomes, undesirable effects, interactions, complications.																																								
Assess if progress toward expected outcomes is being met; makes changes as appropriate.																																								
Trend for Potential Complications																																								
Seeks guidance as appropriate.																																								
Notifies instructor/nurse re: trends /changes in client condition, complications with meds and/or post-procedure & intervene as appropriate.																																								
Yes- You Manage Care to Reduce "RISKS"																																								
Discuss appropriate management activities to include: delegation, room assign, equipment safety, etc. for specific client's needs.																																								
Maintains client safety (fall prevention, bed position, call light, infection control, equipment etc).																																								

Page 2

109

APPENDIX B

CLINICAL EVALUATION TOOL (cont'd)

Clinical Evaluation Tool Using "SAFETY" Model

Student Name:

Clinical Date:

Rating columns (repeated per clinical date): S | NI | U | S | NI | U | S | NI | U | S | NI | U | S | NI | U ... — **Mid-Term** (S | NI | U | NA) — **Final** (S | NI | U | NA)

PERFORMANCE OUTCOMES
Communication
Written & computer charting complete, timely & cosigned by end of shift. Demonstrates ability to use Inform systems technology.
Uses theraupeutic communication techniques.
Non-verbal communication: Aware of importance & impact.
Gives concise, accurate, complete report at end of day following SBAR before leaving assigned unit.
Client teaching concise, accurate; includes health promotion & plan for transitional care.
Professional Behavior
Integrates standards of care, scope of practice, ethical & cultural practice into client care.
Coordinates/collaborates/advocates with interdisciplinary team.
Accepts constructive criticism.
Maintains client/institutional confidentiality, i.e., HIPAA.
Assertive in seeking learning experiences.
Respectful of clients personnel; manages conflict.
Reports on time to unit/conferences & uses spare time constructively.
Adheres to Core Values/handbook/syllabus.
Follows school dress code as outlined in handbook/syllabus.

CLINICAL EVALUATION TOOL *(cont'd)*

Student Name:

Clinical Date:

Clinical Evaluation Tool Using "SAFETY" Model

PERFORMANCE OUTCOMES	Mid-Term																Final			
	S	NI	U	NA	S	NI	U	S	NI	U	S	NI	U	S	NI	U	S	NI	U	NA

Concept Map

Written concept map, w/system-spec assess, priority interventions, eval. of client response & progress toward outcomes, patho page, 2 AIDES sheets & Reflection Questions.

Paperwork turned in on time.

Faculty/student initials

S: Satisfactory; NI: Needs Improvement; U: Unsatisfactory; NA: Not experienced

S: Clinical behavior is safe & demonstrates growth toward course competencies.

NI: Clinical behavior is safe, however, performance is deficient in essential background knowledge.

U: Clinical behavior is unsafe. Performance seldom demonstrates essential knowledge & growth toward competencies.

NA: Clinical behavior not relevant to assigned client.

Absences _____ Late arrivals _____

Faculty _____ Date _____

Student _____ Date _____

Final Clinical Grade _____

Comments:

Page 4

111

APPENDIX C

STAR COUNSELING FORM

Faculty Name: _____   Date of Incident: _____

Student Name: _____   Date of Session: _____

S – SITUATION: Describe the situation.

T – TASK: Requirements and/or policy performance standards that are not being met. (Standards and evaluation criteria published in course syllabus and/or in the University or College of Nursing student handbooks). State reference with page number(s) if applicable.

A – ACTIONS: Plan to improve unsatisfactory performance.

Consequences: Consequences of not meeting performance improvement plan.

R – RESULTS: Date: (Results from actions listed above)

DATE TO IMPROVE PERFORMANCE BY:

Faculty Signature: _____   Date: _____

Student Signature: _____   Date: _____

Observer Signature: _____   Date: _____

EXAMPLE STAR COUNSELING FORM

Faculty Name: <u>Professor Clinical</u>   Date of Incident: <u>January 12, 2018</u>

Student Name: <u>Minnie Student</u>   Date of Session: <u>January 17, 2018</u>

S – SITUATION: Describe the situation:

1. Wore brown shoes to clinical. Stated it was because she had washed her shoes and they were not dry.
2. When asked where her stethoscope was, as she was getting ready for her assessment, she reported it was in the conference room.
3. Conducted an equipment check at the end of clinical and she did not have stethoscope or watch.

T – TASK: Requirements and/or policy performance standards that are not being met. (Safety standards and evaluation criteria published in course syllabus.) State reference with page number(s).

Reference: Course Syllabus. Page 8: Clinical Preparation & Dress Code

Page 11: Statement of Academic Responsibility and clinical orientation

Evaluation Criteria: Ethical behavior

A – ACTIONS: Steps to be taken to improve unsatisfactory performance:

1. Come to clinical in appropriate clinical uniform with white shoes.
2. Bring all equipment needed, stethoscope, watch, scissors, and protective eyewear.
3. Answer questions honestly.

Consequences: Consequences of not meeting performance improvement plan:

Failure to wear correct uniform and bring equipment to clinical will result in being sent home from clinical with a clinical day failure.

Date to improve performance by: Begin immediately with next clinical day, January 19, 2018

Faculty Signature: *Professor Clinical*   Student Signature: *Minnie Student*

Observer Signature: *Professor Lab*

R – RESULTS: Date: (Results from action listed above)

1. Came appropriately dressed for clinical.
2. Had equipment needed for clinical.
3. No further incidents of dishonesty.

FURTHER ACTION NEEDED (none, further counseling, consequences imposed):

No further action needed

Faculty Signature: *Professor Clinical*   Student Signature: *Minnie Student*

Observer Signature: *Professor Lab*

ENGAGING THE LEARNER ACTIVITIES

STUDENT-CENTERED LEARNING ACTIVITIES
LINKED TO PROFESSIONAL AND NCLEX® STANDARDS

Resources Needed for Activity	*The Eight-Step Approach for Student Clinical Success* (Zager, Manning & Herman, 2018)
Standards	**Student Instructions**

Psychosocial Integrity
Manage conflict among clients and healthcare staff.
 	
Physiological Integrity; Basic Care
Monitor client's hydration status.
	Professional Behavior:
	Conflict Management
	(Refer to Clinical Evaluation Tool, Appendix B)
	
	Choose a partner to work with and answer the questions. Your instructor will give you a brief scenario of a conflict between students about the care of a client with fluid volume deficit.
	
	1. Your client has a fluid volume imbalance.
	
	   a. 1st student assess the VS and notes VS are not within normal range. You want to check the VS again in an hour instead of reporting the change now.
	
	   b. 2nd student you want to report the abnormal VS now because the expectation is to report changes in VS to the nurse and/or instructor. You are concerned about potential complications.
	
	   c. **Answer the questions:**
	     1. What are the practice standards?
	     2. What are the potential complications based on the assessed VS and the client's diagnosis?
	     3. What steps could you take when you disagree with your colleague on the plan of care?
	     4. What happens if you take no action?
	     5. What happens if the 2nd student reports the VS even if the 1st student does not agree?
	
	   d. What is the most appropriate decision?

Linking Clinical Experience to NCLEX® Success

> ## IN THIS CHAPTER YOU WILL LEARN HOW TO:
>
> ➤ Apply NCLEX® standards throughout the clinical experience
>
> ➤ Link the "SAFETY" Model to client care to assist in mastering clinical decision making

APPLY NCLEX® STANDARDS THROUGHOUT THE CLINICAL EXPERIENCE

The purpose of the NCLEX-RN® is to ensure safety and welfare of the public (NCSBN, 2018). The exam evaluates specific competencies necessary for the newly licensed, entry-level registered nurse to perform safe and effective care. The NCLEX-RN® Test Plan provides an abbreviated summary of the content and scope of the licensing examination. The Test Plan can be downloaded from the National Council of State Boards of Nursing's website (www.ncsbn.org).

Linking NCLEX-RN® Test Plan activities to the clinical experience is a powerful strategy to use. Regardless who your client is, the NCLEX® standards apply. NCLEX® standards, called activities, reflect patient safety and practice standards. We organized the priority NCLEX® activities/standards in three mnemonics: "**SAFETY**" (Appendix A), "**RISK**" (Appendix B), and "**AIDES**" (Appendix C) to provide you structures for clinical.

The National Council of State Boards of Nursing is moving forward with the Next Generation NCLEX® (NGN) project. The focus is to develop exam item prototypes that measure clinical judgment (NCSBN, 2018). The "SAFETY" model discussed in this chapter provides you a framework for critical thinking and decision making that leads to clinical judgments.

LINK THE "SAFETY" MODEL TO CLINICAL DECISION MAKING

We will show you how to apply the mnemonic "SAFETY" to link standards to client care. The S in "SAFETY" represents both System-Specific Pathophysiology and System-Specific Assessments. System-Specific Pathophysiology tells you what is taking place with the client. If you are caring for a child with frequent swallowing after a tonsillectomy due to bleeding or a post partum client with retained placenta fragments, or a client with a bleeding peptic ulcer, all will have the same physiological changes of bleeding. These physiological changes include an increase in the heart rate, respiratory rate, change in the skin color, and a decrease in temperature, blood pressure, and urine output. Recognizing these signs and symptoms from bleeding are essential for you to prioritize appropriate interventions and prevent potential complications.

What we just described reflects the NCLEX® activities listed below and also are very important patient safety standards:

✔ Identify pathophysiology related to an acute or chronic condition (i.e., signs and symptoms).

✔ Assess and respond to changes in vital signs.

System-Specific Assessment, part of the S in "SAFETY", is another NCLEX® activity/standard. You need to know how to complete a fast system-specific assessment with a focus on the presenting symptoms versus a detailed one-hour head-to-toe assessment. You should begin your assessment the minute you walk into the client's room.

Using the above example of bleeding, connect the similarities and/or differences in both the system-specific assessments and the TRENDS with the hemodynamic changes that may occur. You need to know early signs of bleeding (i.e., increased heart rate, respiratory rate, etc.) versus the late signs and symptoms of bleeding (i.e., decreased blood pressure and urine output, etc.) so you can intervene early to prevent potential complications. We now have discussed four additional NCLEX® activities/standards under system-specific assessments:

✔ Perform focused assessment and re-assessment.

✔ Assess and respond to changes in vital signs.

✔ Recognize signs and symptoms of complications and intervene appropriately when providing care.

✔ Recognize trends and changes in client condition and intervene.

System-specific labs and diagnostic procedures are also part of the system-specific assessments. Analyzing lab values and performing diagnostic tests (i.e., EKG, O_2 saturation, glucose monitoring, etc.) gives you additional information needed for clinical decision making. Develop the habit of reviewing lab values and linking the significance of these to your client's nursing care. We have included a **Lab and Diagnostic Tests and Procedures Tool** in Chapter 4 (Appendix H).

Specific information regarding these can be reviewed in the book *Nursing Made Insanely Easy* by Manning & Rayfield (2016). The following mnemonic "**DIAGNOSTIC**" reflects the pertinent NCLEX® activities:

D iagnostic test results—monitor; intervene for complications.

I njury and/or complications from procedure should be prevented.

A ssist with invasive procedures (e.g., thoracentesis, bronchoscopy).

G lucose monitoring, ECG, O_2 saturation, etc. may be performed.

N ote client's response to procedures and treatments.

O btain specimens other than blood (e.g., wound, stool, etc.).

S igns and symptoms of trends and/or changes-monitor, and intervene.

T each client and family about procedures and treatments.

I dentify vital signs and monitor for changes and intervene.

C omplications should be noted and followed immediately with an action.

The **A** in "SAFETY" represents **Analyzing priority nursing concepts** based on the system-specific assessments. After assessing your client and determining the concepts that apply to your client, prioritize the care. If you are unsure of the priority of care for your client, ask your clinical instructor to assist you. The NCLEX® activity/standard is:

✔ Assess/triage clients to prioritize order of care delivery.

The **F** in "SAFETY" represents both nursing interventions that should be implemented **First** as well as medications that should be administered **First**. When the client has four nursing interventions in need of implementation, ask yourself these questions: *"What are the priority nursing actions? Which client needs immediate nursing action and why? What medications should be administered first for specific clinical assessments?"*

For example, if a client begins expectorating blood and is in the supine position, then the priority nursing action would be for you to reposition client. This would be done even prior to notifying the healthcare provider or initiating a complete assessment. If you have two clients bleeding, review the trends in the vital signs, I & O, and/or LOC to assist in identifying early or late signs of bleeding to determine which client to see first.

Another example is a client with respiratory problems who has an order to administer a corticosteroid inhaler and a Beta$_2$ Adrenergic Agonist such as Albuterol. Connect the actions for both of these drugs with the pathophysiology to understand the rationale for administering Albuterol prior to the steroid inhaler. This reflects the NCLEX® activity/standard:

✔ Prioritize the delivery of client care.

The **E** in "SAFETY" will assist you to remember to **Evaluate the Expected Outcomes** from the nursing care as well as from the medications. The **Evaluation of Expected Outcomes** provides the information you need to make clinical judgments about the plan of care. Review the process of evaluation of expected outcomes (Refer to Chapter 4, p. 57–58). These evaluations might include:

✦ Did the bleeding stop?

✦ Did the breath sounds improve?

✦ Did the vital signs return to baseline?

✦ Did the medication assist in reducing the intracranial pressure?

✦ Did the medication assist in reducing the serum glucose?

The NCLEX® activities addressed include:

✔ Evaluate/document response to treatment.

✔ Evaluate therapeutic effect of medications.

The **T** in "SAFETY," **Trend for Potential Complications**, reminds you to consistently compare and contrast vital signs, I & O, neurological assessments, drainage, etc. as part of your clinical assessment. For a complete review of trends to monitor for preventing complications, refer to the book *Nursing Made Insanely Easy* (Manning & Rayfield, 2016, p. 8–9). As you become more proficient with trending, begin to organize the assessments into early versus late clinical findings. If the client is unstable and presenting with late signs and symptoms, it is imperative for you to intervene with priority intervention(s) to prevent the client from deteriorating and experiencing a crisis.

An example of trends would be a client who is receiving the drug magnesium sulfate. The urine output had been 85 mL/hour, and the next hour the urine output is 45 mL/hour. It is imperative to report the trend of the decreasing urine output immediately because magnesium sulfate is excreted in the urine. You do not wait for the urine output to continue to decline even though 45 mL/hr is within normal range. If you need assistance and support to make your clinical decision, work with your clinical instructor. The NCLEX® activities/standards represent the Client Need Category of Reduction of Risk and are reviewed below:

✔ Recognize trends and changes in client condition and intervene.

✔ Recognize signs and symptoms of complications and intervene appropriately when providing care.

✔ Assess and respond to changes in vital signs.

The **Y** in "SAFETY" stands for **You Must Manage Care to Prevent "RISK" to the client**. "RISK" is a mnemonic that will help you know what to assess and how to manage care to prevent "RISKS."

R   Room Assignments, **R**ecognize limitations of staff, **R**estraint safety, **R**isk for falls, **R**eceive or give report

I   Identify trends, **I**nfection control, **I**dentification of client, **I**dentify accuracy of orders, **I**nformed consent, **I**nterdisciplinary Team Collaboration

S   Skin breakdown, **S**afe equipment, **S**cope of Practice for delegation

K   Know Standards of Practice, **K**now how to document, **K**now how to prepare for transfer, discharge, **K**now how to teach and incorporate health-promotion standards

Your clinical instructor may ask you to complete "**RISK**" (Appendix B) for your client. "**RISK**" will help you focus on client safety during clinical.

The mnemonic "**AIDES**" (Appendix C) is a structure for organizing the NCLEX® activities/ standards that focus on pharmacology. This is a great tool you can use throughout your curriculum for you to be successful regarding pharmacology with your clients and on the NCLEX®.

These three mnemonics "**SAFETY**" (Appendix A), "**AIDES**" (Appendix B), and "**RISK**" (Appendix C) provide a structure to link NCLEX® activities/standards while caring for your clients.

SAFETY

This structure can help prioritize NCLEX® activities that can be evaluated through the **Concept Map**, **AIDES**, **Reflection Questions**, and **History and Pathophysiology Assessment Tool** (refer to Chapter 4 (Appendices C, D, E, and G).

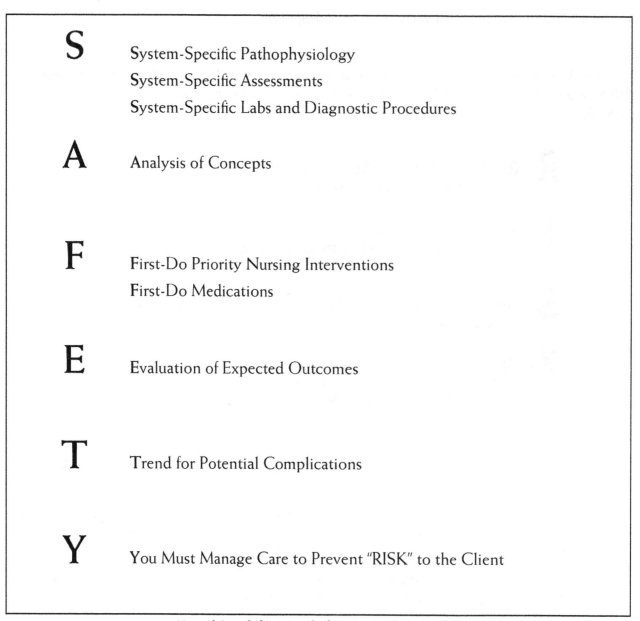

S	System-Specific Pathophysiology
	System-Specific Assessments
	System-Specific Labs and Diagnostic Procedures
A	Analysis of Concepts
F	First-Do Priority Nursing Interventions
	First-Do Medications
E	Evaluation of Expected Outcomes
T	Trend for Potential Complications
Y	You Must Manage Care to Prevent "RISK" to the Client

National Council of State Boards of Nursing, Inc. (NCSBN) 2018

RISK

A structure for prioritizing Management and Safety NCLEX® Activities. Directions: *Please complete on your client assignment. Turn in to clinical instructor* _____.

R   Room Assignments, Recognize limitations of staff, Restraint safety, Risk for falls, Receive or give report

I   Identify trends, Infection control, Identification of client, Identify accuracy of orders, Informed consent, Interdisciplinary Team Collaboration

S   Skin breakdown, Safe equipment, Scope of Practice for delegation

K   Know Standards of Practice, Know how to document, Know how to prepare for transfer, discharge, Know how to teach and incorporate health-promotion standards

National Council of State Boards of Nursing, Inc. (NCSBN) 2018

AIDES

A structure for prioritizing Pharmacology NCLEX® Activities. Directions: *Please complete on ___ of your priority medications. Turn in to clinical instructor _____.*

NAME OF DRUG: BRAND _____ GENERIC _____

CLASSIFICATION: _____ REFERENCE USED _____

A	Action of medication:
	Administration of medication. Dosage ordered_____
	How to administer:
	Assessment:
	Adverse Effects. List significant ones:
	Accuracy/Appropriateness of order. Is it indicated based on client's condition, known allergies, drug-drug or drug-food interactions? If not, what action did you take?
I	Interactions (Drug-Drug, Food-Drug):
	Identify priority plan prior to giving drug (i.e., vital signs, labs, allergies, etc.):
	Identify priority plan after giving drug:
D	Desired outcomes of the drug:
	Discharge teaching—Administration considerations for client and family:
	Documentation:
E	Evaluate client's response to medication:
S	Safety (client identification, risk for falls, vital sign assessments):
	Safe and controlled environment for handling and maintaining medicine:

National Council of State Boards of Nursing, Inc. (NCSBN) 2018

ENGAGING THE LEARNER ACTIVITIES

STUDENT-CENTERED LEARNING ACTIVITIES
LINKED TO PROFESSIONAL AND NCLEX® STANDARDS

Resources Needed for Activities	*Concepts Made Insanely Easy for Clinical Nursing* (Manning & Zager, 2014);*The Eight-Step Approach for Student Clinical Success* (Zager, Manning & Herman, 2018); *Medical Surgical Nursing Concepts Made Insanely Easy* (Manning & Zager, 2014)
Standards	**Student Instructions**

Management of Care
 	
Prioritize the delivery of client care.
	Trending for Potential Complications
	
	1. Based on your assigned client, what are the potential complications?
	
	   a. What system-specific assessments would be a priority?
	
	   b. If you see a trend, what other assessments would provide additional information?
	
	   c. What are the trends in the clinical findings?
	
	   d. Compare and contrast the findings to the clinical norms or the client's normal.
	
	   e. What clinical findings would need to be reported to the assigned nurse and/or the healthcare provider?

Safe and Effective Care Environment
 	
Apply principles of infection control (i.e., hand hygiene, room assignment, isolation, etc.).
	RISK to the Client—Infection Control
	(Refer to Chapter 23, *Medical Surgical Nursing Concepts Made Insanely Easy*)
	
	2. Based on the clients:
	
	   a. Choose the personal protective equipment (PPE) needed for the care you will provide to your client indicated on the index card.
	
	   b. Choose which two of your four clients indicated on the index cards can share a room: a client post-op appendectomy with MRSA, a client with hospital acquired C. diff, a client admitted with hepatitis, or a client with MRSA from a traumatic injury to the right leg?

NOTES

References

Agency for Healthcare Research and Quality (AHRQ). Retrieved from http://www.ahrq.gov/, November 10, 2016.

Agency for Healthcare Research and Quality (2015). Medication errors. Retrieved from https://psnet.ahrq.gov/primers/primer/23/medication-errorsc.

Beyea, S. (2014). Interruptions and distractions in health care: Improved safety with mindfulness. Retrieved from https://psnet.ahrq.gov/perspectives/perspective/152/.

Blum, C.A., Borglund, S., & Parcells, D. (2010). High-fidelity nursing simulation: Impact on student self-confidence and clinical competence. *International Journal of Nursing Education Scholarship*, 7(article 18), Retrieved from https://www.ncbi.nlm.nih.gov/pubmed/20597857.

Cannon, S. & Boswell, C. (Eds.) (2016). Evidence-based teaching in nursing: A foundation for educators, (2nd ed.). Burlington, MA: Jones & Bartlett.

Center for Disease Control (2015). Growth chart training. Retrieved from http://www.cdc.gov/nccdphp/dnpao/growthcharts/.

Dreifuerst, K.T. (2009). The essentials of debriefing in simulation learning: A concept analysis. Nursing Education Perspectives. 30(2), 109-114.

Dreifuerst, K.T. (2012). Using debriefing for meaning learning to foster development of clinical reasoning in simulation. Journal of Nursing Education. June 51(6), 326-333.

Griggs, J. (2017). Generational Learning Styles (Generation X and Y). Retrieved from http://web2.fit.edu/ctle/documents/Webinar_Handouts/Generational%20Learning%20Styles%20Handout.pdf, July 23, 2017.

Hayden, J.K., Smiley, R.A., Alexander, M., Kardong-Edgren, S., & Jeffries, P.R. (2014). The NCSBN national simulation study: A longitudinal, randomized, controlled study replacing clinical hours with simulation in prelicensure nursing education. *Journal of Nursing Regulation*. 5, 1–66.

Herman, J. W. (2008). Creative teaching strategies for the nurse educator. Philadelphia, PA: F.A. Davis Company.

Hughes, R.G. (Ed) (2008). Patient Safety & Quality: An evidence-based handbook for nurses. (Prepared with support from the Robert Wood Johnson Foundation.) AHRQ Publication No. 08-0043. Rockville, MD: Agency for Healthcare Research and Quality; April 2008.

Institute for Healthcare Improvement (2018). SBAR tool: Situation-Background-Assessment-Evaluation. Retrieved from http://www.ihi.org/resources/Pages/Tools/SBARToolkit.aspx

Institute for Safe Medication (ISMP). Retrieved from http://www.ismp.org/, November 16, 2016.

International Nursing Association for Clinical Simulation and Learning (INACSL). INACSL Standards of Best Practice: SimulationSM. Retrieved from http://www.inacsl.org/i4a/pages/index.cfm?pageid=3407, November 8, 2016.

Jefferies, P.R. & Clochesy, J.M. (2012). Clinical simulations: An experiential, student-centered pedagogical approach. In D. M. Billings and J.A. Halstead (Eds). Teaching in nursing: A guide for faculty (4th ed., pp 352-368). St. Louis, MO: Elsevier Health Sciences.

Jefferies, P.R., Dreifuerst, K.T., Kardon-Edgren, S., & Hayden, J. (2015). Faculty development when initialing simulation programs: Lessons learned from the National Simulation Study. Journal of Nursing Regulation, 5(4), 17-23.

Jefferies, P.R. & Rogers, K.J. (2002). Theoretical framework for simulation design. In P.R. Jeffries (Ed.), Simulation in nursing education: From conceptualization to evaluation (2nd ed., pp 25-41). New York, NY: National League for Nursing.

Kaufer, D. (2016). Neuroscience and how students learn. Graduate Student Instructor Teaching and Resource Center, How Students Learn Series, University of California Berkley. Retrieved from http://gsi.berkeley.edu/gsi-guide-contents/learning-theory-research/neuroscience .

Koharchnik, L. (2014). Starting a job as adjunct clinical instructor. American Journal of Nursing, 114(8), p. 57-60.

Koharchnik, L, Caputi, L., Robb, M., & Culleiton, A. L. (2015). Fostering clinical reasoning in nursing students (2015). American Journal of Nursing, 115(1), 58-61.

Koharchnik, L, Weideman, Y. L., Walters, C. A., & Hardy, E. (2015). Evaluating nursing students' clinical performance. American Journal of Nursing, 115(10), 64-67.

Levett-Jones, T., Hoffman, K., Dempsey, J., Jeong, S., Noble, D., Norton, C., Roche, J., & Hickey, N. (2009). The 'five rights' of clinical reasoning: An educational model to enhance nursing students' ability to identify and manage clinically 'at risk' patients. Nurse Educator Today, 30, 515-520.

Lioce L., Meakim, C.H., Fey, M.K., Chmil, J.V., Mariani, B., & Alinier, G. (2015). Standards of best practice: Simulation standard IX: Simulation design. Clinical Simulation in Nursing, 11(6), 309-315, Retrieved from http://dx.doi.org/10.1016/j.ecns.2015.03.005.

Manning, L. & Rayfield, S. (2016). Nursing made insanely easy, Duluth, GA: ICAN Publishing, Inc.

Manning, L. & Rayfield, S. (2017). Pharmacology made insanely easy. Duluth, GA: ICAN Publishing, Inc.

Manning, L. & Zager, L. (2014). Concepts made insanely easy for clinical nursing. Duluth, GA: ICAN Publishing, Inc.

Manning, L. & Zager, L. (2014). Medical surgical nursing concepts made insanely easy! A new approach to prioritization, Duluth, GA: ICAN Publishing, Inc.

Meakim, C., Boese, T., Decker, S., Franklin, A. E., Gloe, D., Lioce, L., Sando, C. R., & Borum, J. C. (2013). Standards of best practice: Simulation standard I: Terminology. *Clinical Simulation in Nursing*, 9(6S), S3-S11, Retrieved from http://dx.doi.org/10.1016/j.ecns.2013.04.001.

Merkel, S. I., Voepel-Lewis, T., Shayevitz, J. R., & Malviya, S. (1997). The FLACC: A behavioral scale for scoring postoperative pain in young children. Pediatric Nursing, 23(3), 293–297.

National Council of State Boards of Nursing. (NCSBN) 2017. RN Practice Analysis: Linking the NCLEX-RN® Examination to practice U.S. and Canada (Volume 72) February 2018.

National Council of State Boards of Nursing, Inc. (2018). NCSBN Research Brief; Strategic Practice Analysis. 71(1).

National Council of State Boards of Nursing, Inc. (2018). Measuring the right things. NCSBN's next generation NCLEX® endeavors to go beyond the leading edge. *In Focus, A publication of the National Council State Boards of Nursing*, 12, Winter.

National League for Nursing Simulation Innovation Resource Center (NLN-SIRC) (2013). SIRC glossary, Retrieved from http://sirc.nln.org/mod/glossary/view.php?id=183&mode=&hook=ALL&sortkey=&sortorder=&fullsearch=0&page=1.

National Patient Safety Goals (2017). 2017 Hospital national patient safety goals. Retrieved from https://www.jointcommission.org/assets/1/6/2017_NPSG_HAP_ER.pdf, January 12, 2017.

Nevid, J. (2011). Teaching the millennials. Retrieved from http://www.psychologicalscience.org/publications/observer/2011/may-june-11/teaching-the-millennials.html.

Oguh, E. (2017). Dispelling common myths about millennials in the workforce. Retrieved from http://www.huffingtonpost.com/entry/dispelling-common-myths-about-millennials-in-the-workforce_us_5973fa93e4b0f1feb89b4410, July 23, 2017.

Penn, B.K. (Ed) (2008). Mastering the teaching role: A guide for nurse educators, Philadelphia, PA: F.A. Davis.

Pesut, D., & Herman, J.A., (1999). Clinical reasoning: The art and science of critical and creative thinking, Albany, NY: Delmar Publishing.

Quality and Safety Education for Nurses (QSEN). Retrieved from http://qsen.org/, November 22, 2016.

Reid, C. & Raleigh, R. (2013). Where to find simulations free. Retrieved from https://www.scribd.com/document/299632811/Where-to-Find-Simulation-Scenarios.

Simulation for Society in Healthcare 2016. Retrieved from http://www.ssih.org/About-Simulation, November 7, 2016.

University of Hawaii System (2017). Effectively teaching generation z. Retrieved from https://www.hawaii.edu/ovppp/Leaders/files/2015-2016-Projects/PELP_GenZ_PaperV.6.0-5.4.16.pdf . July 23, 2017.

Walls, C. (2006). The multitasking generation. Retrieved from http://www.time.com/time/archive/preview/0,10987,1174696,00.html.

Waxman, K. T. (2010). The development of evidence-based clinical simulation scenarios: Guidelines for nurse educators. *Journal of Nursing Education*, 49(1), 29-35.

Williams, A. (2015). Move over, millennials, here comes generation Z. Retrieved from http://www.nytimes.com/2015/09/20/fashion/move-over-millennials-here-comes-generation-z.html?_r=0.

World Health Organiztion (2010). National Center for Growth Statistics. Retrieved from https://cdc.gov/growthcharts/index.htm.

Zager, L., Manning, L. & Herman, J. (2017). The eight-step approach to teaching clinical nursing. Duluth, GA: ICAN Publishing, Inc.

URLs for Simulation Scenarios, References and Scenario Design

http://www.sim-central.com/documents/scenarios.pdf

http://healthysimulation.com/5689/free-medical-simulation-scenarios/

http://healthysimulation.com/1947/more-free-nursing-simulation-scenarios/

http://sirc.nln.org/login/index.php

http://www.ksbn.org/education/Scenario/SimulationScenarioLibrary.htm

http://qsen.org/teaching-strategies/simulation/scenarios/

http://www.nursingsimulation.org/article/S1876-1399(15)00025-0/references

Index

A

Active learning (*see* Engaging the Learner Activities)
Adult health concept map example, 61–62
   rubric grading tool, 63
   concept map tool, 64–65
AIDES, 122
AIDES Medication Information Tool, 66
Algorithm, urinary catheterization, 31, 42
   procedure template, 43
Analyzing priority nursing concepts, 32, 34–35, 61–63, 75–76, 117
Assess readiness to be a clinical nursing
   student, 1, 5–6
Assessments, system specific, 32–34, 52–53, 61–63, 116

B

Black box warnings (BBW), 21

C

Call to healthcare provider example, SBAR, 24
Cardiac/peripheral perfusion,
   assessments, system-specific, 76, 80
   concept, 82
   interventions, first-do priority, 76–77, 81
   outcomes, expected, 77, 82
   pathophysiology, 79
Clinical day,
   how to structure, 11, 14–17
   typical day schedule, student guide 18
   template typical schedule, student guide, 19
Change of shift report example, SBAR, 22
Clinical evaluation, 101–114
   criteria for, 101–102

evaluation tool, 108–111
   participating in evaluation process, 104–105
Clinical decision making, 27–28, 30–31, 47, 116–119
   Improving clinical decision making, 27–31
Clinical decision making thinking strategies, 44–45
   knowledge work, 44
   prototype identification, 44
   hypothesizing, 44
   self-talk, 44
   schema search, 44
   if–then thinking, 45
   compare and contrast, 45
   trending, 45
Clinical findings, structure and organize, 12
Clinical judgments, 27, 33, 54, 57–58, 62, 65
Clinical reasoning, 27
Clinical self-assessment questionnaire, 5–6
COACH, learning success strategies, 3–4
Concepts,
   relationships among the concepts, 50–51
   mastering, 75–78
   oxygenation, 83–86
   perfusion, cardiac and peripheral, 79–82
   prioritizing, 77–78
Concept map, 47–60, 104
   adult health concept map example, 61–62
   grading rubric, 63
   how to construct and use, 48–60
   using in clinical practice, 59
Concept map tool, 64–65
Compare and contrast in clinical decision making, 45
Comparison of basic assessments with trending for potential complications, 28–29

Complications, trend for potential, 28–29, 39, 53, 118–119
Counseling session, 105–106
   STAR counseling form, 112
   STAR counseling example, 113
Critical thinking, 27
Criteria, clinical evaluation, 101–102

D

Debriefing for meaningful learning (DML), 94
   Receive and participate, 94
Decision making, clinical thinking strategies, 44–46
   knowledge work, 44
   prototype identification, 44
   hypothesizing, 44
   self-talk, 44
   schema search, 44
   if–then thinking, 45
   compare and contrast, 45
   trending, 45
Decision making, 27–28, 30
Decision making, linked to SAFETY model, 116–119
Determine Outcomes and Evaluation Criteria Table, 54
Developing Outcomes and Evaluation Criteria with Interventions, 56
Develop prioritization strategies, 27–28
Diagnostic tests/procedures, 34, 73
Documentation, 5, 15, 18–19, 37–38, 40, 59

E

Engaging the Learner Activities, 9, 25, 46, 74, 87, 99, 100, 114, 123
Evaluate expected outcomes, 32, 38–39, 62–63, 77, 118
Evaluation, participating in, 104–105
Evaluation, unsafe care practices, 102
Evaluation concept map criteria table, 54

F

Feedback, 101–103
   Using feedback effectively,
     102–103
First-do priority interventions, 32–33,
   35–38, 55–56, 61–63, 117–118

G

Generational learning differences
   characteristics, 3, 9
   Generation X, 3
   Generation Y–Millennials, 3
   Generation Z, 3
   Multi-generational learner, 9
Guide, student typical day schedule,
   18
Guide, student typical day template,
   19

H

Health history and system-specific
   assessment tool, 68–70
Helpful tips when preparing for
   simulation, 95
High fidelity manikins, 89
High-stakes simulation, 90
History and pathophysiology
   information tool, 68
Hypothesizing, 44, 49

I

If-then thinking in clinical decision
   making, 45
Inquiry questions, 27, 30–31, 35–40,
   53, 58
   examples of, 44–45
Inquiry questions for classroom
   organized around the "safety"
   model, 34–40
   types of, 31
Inquiry questions for a urinary
   catheterization procedure, 42
Interactive clinical learning strategies,
   7–8
Interrelationships among concepts,
   50–51
Interventions, priority, 55–56, 77–78,
   117–118

J

Judgment, 27
   Judgment of evaluation of clinical
     outcomes, 33, 54, 57–58, 62, 65
   plan of care, 57–58

K

Knowledge work, 44

L

Lab and diagnostic tests, 34, 116–117
   procedures tool, 71–73
Learning strategies,
   interactive clinical, 4, 7–8
Learning styles, 1–2
   generational characteristics, 3
   success strategies for learning, 3–4
Linking pathophysiology to
   first-do priority interventions for
     altered oxygenation, 85
   first-do priority interventions for
     cardiac/ peripheral perfusion, 81
   system-specific assessments for
     altered oxygenation, 84
   system-specific assessments for
     cardiac and peripheral perfusion,
     80
Low-stakes simulation, 90

M

Manikins,
   high fidelity, 89
   high-stakes simulation, 90
   low fidelity, 90
   low-stakes simulation, 90
   moderate or mid-fidelity, 90
Medication administration, 12, 21,
   36–38 ,40
   7 rights of, 102
   protocol: a safe approach, 12, 21,
     25
   medication information tool, 66,
     122
   multi-generational learner, 3, 9

N

National Council of State Boards of
   Nursing,
     Applying standards, 115–122
     standards, 78, 104
NCLEX-RN® test plan, 115
Negative feedback, 102–103
Neural networks, 1
Novice students, 2
Nursing concepts analyzing, 117
Nursing concept maps, 47–60
   example of an adult health concept
     map, 61–62
   example of an adult health concept
     map grading tool (rubric), 63
   example of an adult health concept
     map tool, 64–65

O

Outcomes and Evaluation Criteria, 54
Outcomes and Evaluation Criteria
   with Interventions, 56
Outcome Not Met, 57

Outcome Partially Achieved, 58
Outcome Achieved, 58
Oxygenation, SAFETY, linking
   pathophysiology to system-specific
   assessments, 84
Oxygenation, SAFETY, linking
   pathophysiology to first-do nursing
   interventions, 85
Oxygenation, SAFETY summary
   concept, 86

P

Pathophysiological process, 76–77
Pathophysiology behind alterations in
   oxygenation, 83–85
Pathophysiology behind decrease in
   cardiac/peripheral perfusion, 79–81
Performance evaluation, 101–106,
   108–111
Perfusion, 75, 82
Physical assessment, 70
Pitfalls of feedback, 102–103
Preparing medications for
   administration, 21
Priority concepts
   analyze, 75–76
   determine priority interventions,
     55, 76–77
   evaluate expected outcomes,
     57–58, 77
   identify related, 50–51, 77–78
Prioritize nursing care: A new
   systematic approach "SAFETY", 33
Procedure algorithm template, 43
Professional behaviors, 102, 104, 110,
   114
Prototype identification in clinical
   decision making, 44

Q

Questionnaire; Clinical Self-
   Assessment, 5–6
Quick Approach: Inquiry Questions
   for Classroom and Clinical, 30,
   34–40

R

Reflection questions
   examples of, 31, 41, 44–45, 67
Reflective thinking, 31
RISK, 32, 33, 39–40, 96, 98, 107, 109,
   115, 119–121, 123
Role-playing, low fidelity simulation,
   90
Rubric grading tool for concept map,
   63

S

Safe Approach, Medication Administration Practices, 21
"SAFETY" model, 32–40, 107–110, 115–120
  analyzing priority nursing concepts, 32–33, 35, 49, 75–76
  analysis: concepts/outcomes, 108
  analysis and connected priority nursing concept, 35
  analysis of concepts, 107
  communication, 110
  evaluation of expected outcomes, 32, 38–39, 107, 109
  first-do plans, 35
  first-do priority intervention, 32, 35–36, 107–108
  first-do priority medications, 36–38
  interventions, 35–36
  procedures, 38
  professional behavior, 110
  studying with the, 107
  system-specific assessments, 32, 34, 52–53, 108
  system-specific labs and diagnostic procedures, 34
  system-specific pathophysiology, 32, 34
  system-specific physiology assessments lab/procedures, 107
  trend potential complications, 32, 39, 107, 109
  you must manage care: prevent "RISKs", 39–40, 107, 109
  you must manage "risk" for the client, 32, 39, 119
SBAR report, 20
SBAR structure, 13
  for call to healthcare provider, 13, 23–24
  for patient handoff at change of shift, 13, 22, 93
  shift report using SBAR format, 20, 22
Scavenger hunt, 7, 9, 99
  Interactive clinical learning activities, 7–8
Schema search in clinical decision making, 44
Self-assessment, 1–2, 5–6
Self-talk in clinical decision making, 44
Seven rights for medication administration, 21
Shift Report Using SBAR format, 20
Simulation components, 89
  debriefing for meaningful learning (DML), 94
  helpful tips, 95
  participating in the simulation, 92–93
  prepare for simulation, 90–92
  preparation tool, 96–98
STAR format for counseling, 105, 112–113
Step by Step approach to constructing and using the concept map, 47–60
Strategies
  Interactive learning, 7–8
Structure Medication Administration, 12
Structures organizing NCLEX® standards
  AIDES, 66, 122
  RISK, 32, 119, 121
  SAFETY, 32, 116–119, 120
  DIAGNOSTIC PROCEDURES, 117
Structure SBAR for different scenarios, 13
Structuring a clinical day, 14–19
Structuring medication administration, 12
Student-Centered Learning Activities, 9, 25, 46, 74, 87, 99–100, 114, 123
Studying with the "SAFETY" Model, 107
System-specific assessments, 34, 76–77, 116
  analysis of, 78
System-specific labs and diagnostic procedures, 116–117
System-specific pathophysiology, 34, 116

T

Task trainers, 90
Template of Typical Day Schedule, 19
Thinking strategies, 28, 31, 44–45
  thinking-beyond-action, 94
  thinking-in-action, 94
  thinking-on-action, 94
  to develop clinical decision making, 31
  to improve clinical judgment, 44–45
    compare & contrast, 45
    hypothesizing, 44
    if-then thinking, 45
    knowledge work, 44
    prototype identification, 44
    schema search, 44
    self-talk, 44
    trending, 45
Tool for clinical evaluation, 108–111
Trends for potential complications, 28–29, 118, 120
Triage, 35, 117
Typical day schedule, a student guide, 18

U

Urinary catheterization algorithm, 42

W

Weekly evaluations, 104–105
Warning counseling form, 104–106

OTHER BOOKS PUBLISHED BY I CAN PUBLISHING®, INC.

The Eight-Step Approach for Student Clinical Success
Medical Surgical Nursing Concepts Made Insanely Easy!
Concepts Made Insanely Easy for Clinical Nursing!
Pharmacology Made Insanely Easy!
Nursing Made Insanely Easy!
NCLEX-RN® 101: How to Pass!
NCLEX-PN® 101: How to Pass!

TEACHING BOOKS & TOOLS FOR NURSING EDUCATORS

The Eight-Step Approach to Teaching Clinical Nursing
Medical Surgical Nursing Made Insanely Easy! Images on CD
Pharmacology Made Insanely Easy! Images on CD
Nursing Made Insanely Easy! Images on CD
Pharmacology Made Insanely Easy! Audio CD Review
Pathways to Teaching Nursing: Keeping It Real!

STUDENT PROGRAMS

Student programs are available to assist nursing students in learning how to remember and apply both pharmacology and medical surgical nursing concepts to clinical, classroom, testing, and NCLEX® SUCCESS.

Nursing Concepts Made Insanely Easy—a one-day workshop designed to make learning Nursing Concepts Insanely Easy! Tools and illustrations are integrated throughout the workshop to facilitate both nursing school and NCLEX® SUCCESS! Students will learn how to think, prioritize, and make clinical decisions.

Tailored workshops, and presentations, designed with you and the authors to meet your individual needs.

I CAN
PUBLISHING® INC.

Contact I CAN Publishing®, Inc. today to schedule your program.

770.495.2488

www.icanpublishing.com

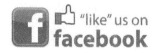